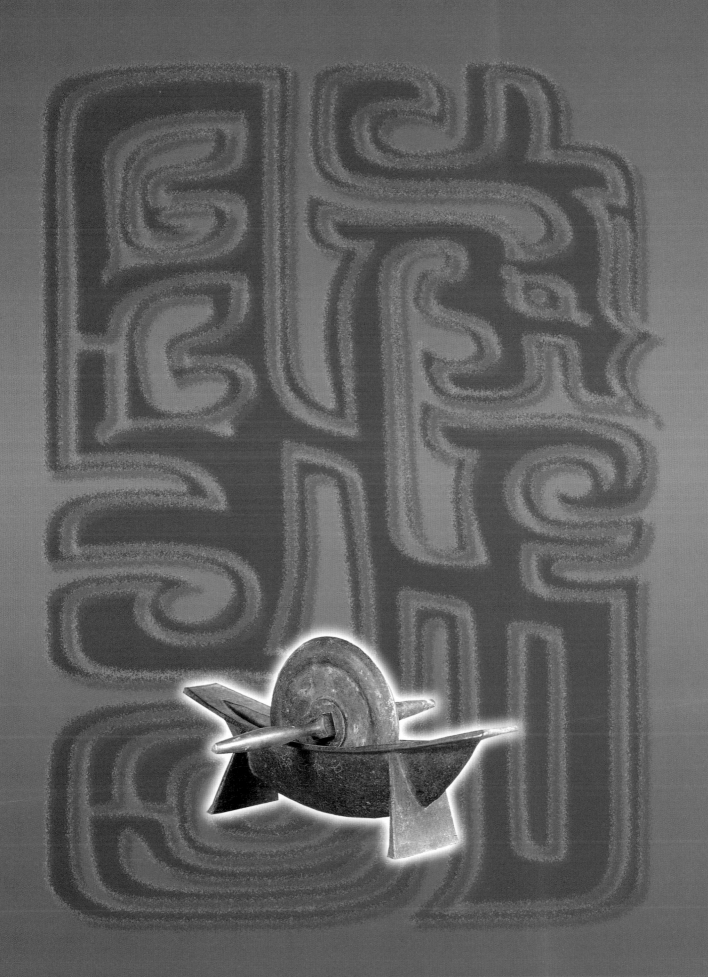

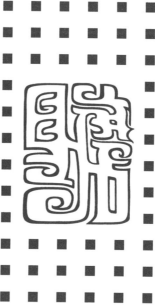

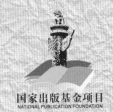

国家出版基金项目
NATIONAL PUBLICATION FOUNDATION

中华医药卫生

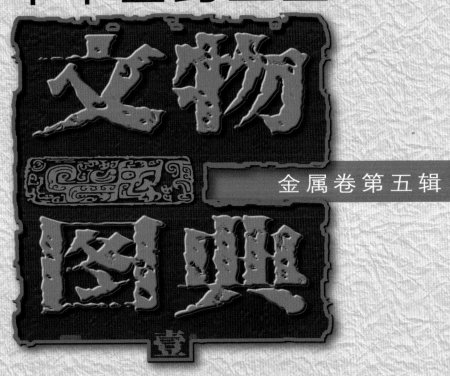

金属卷第五辑

主　编　李经纬　梁　峻　刘学春
总主译　白永权
主　译　吉　乐

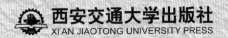

西安交通大学出版社
XI'AN JIAOTONG UNIVERSITY PRESS

图书在版编目（CIP）数据

中华医药卫生文物图典 . 1. 金属卷 . 第 5 辑 . / 李经纬，

梁峻，刘学春主编 . — 西安：西安交通大学出版社，2016.12

ISBN 978-7-5605-7027-3

Ⅰ . ①中… Ⅱ . ①李… ②梁… ③刘… Ⅲ . ①中国医药学—

金属器物—古器物—中国—图录 Ⅳ . ① R-092 ② K870.2

中国版本图书馆 CIP 数据核字（2015）第 013561 号

书　　名　中华医药卫生文物图典（一）金属卷第五辑

主　　编　李经纬　梁　峻　刘学春

责任编辑　李　晶

出版发行　西安交通大学出版社

　　　　　（西安市兴庆南路 10 号　邮政编码 710049）

网　　址　http://www.xjtupress.com

电　　话　（029）82668805　82668502（医学分社）

　　　　　（029）82668315（总编办）

传　　真　（029）82668280

印　　刷　中煤地西安地图制印有限公司

开　　本　889mm×1194mm　1/16　印张 31.25　字数 470 千字

版次印次　2017 年 12 月第 1 版　2017 年 12 月第 1 次印刷

书　　号　ISBN 978-7-5605-7027-3

定　　价　980.00 元

读者购书、书店添货、如发现印装质量问题，请通过以下方式联系、调换。

订购热线：（029）82665248　（029）82665249

投稿热线：（029）82668805　（029）82668502

读者信箱：medpress@126.com

铭记感受历史
自信自重自强自强

中华医药卫生文物图典问世
书贺

陈可冀 谨题
二〇一七年青

陈可冀　中国科学院院士、国医大师

精修醫藥衛生文物

圖典功著當代

深究岐黃學術思想

渊源惠澤千秋

中華醫藥衛生文物圖典出版志慶

丁酉孟秋 孫光荣 敬題於北京

孙光荣　国医大师

中華醫藥衛生文物圖典出版

彰顯中醫藥
文化精神

體現中醫藥
歷史價值

歲次丁酉夏　王琦

王琦　国医大师

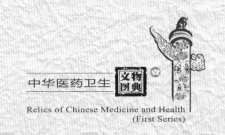

中华医药卫生文物图典（First Series）

中华医药卫生文物图典（一）
丛书编撰委员会

主　编　李经纬　梁　峻　刘学春

副主编　廖　果　吴鸿洲　康兴军　和中浚　刘小斌　杨金生
　　　　郑怀林　徐江雁　白建疆　黄　煌

编　委　李洪晓　梁永宣　王强虎　董树平　马　健　王　霞
　　　　张雅宗　朱德明　包哈申　张建青　郑　蓉　庄乾竹
　　　　李宏红　刘哲峰　王宏才　陈润东

总主译　白永权

主　译　陈向京　聂文信　范晓晖　温　睿　赵永生　杜彦龙
　　　　吉　乐　李小棉　郭　梦　陈　曦

副主译（按姓氏音序排列）
　　　　董艳云　姜雨孜　李建西　刘　慧　马　健　任宝磊
　　　　任　萌　任　莹　王　颇　习通源　谢皖吉　徐素云
　　　　许崇钰　许　梅　詹菊红　赵　菲　邹郝晶

译　者（按姓氏音序排列）

迟征宇　邓　甜　付一豪　高　琛　高　媛　郭　宁

韩　蕾　何宗昌　胡勇强　黄　鋆　蒋新蕾　康晓薇

李静波　刘雅恬　刘妍萌　鲁显生　马　月　牛笑语

唐云鹏　唐臻娜　田　多　铁红玲　佟健一　王　晨

王　丹　王　栋　王　丽　王　媛　王慧敏　王梦杰

王仙先　吴耀均　席　慧　肖国强　许子洋　闫红贤

杨姣姣　姚　晔　张　阳　张　鋆　张继飞　张梦原

张晓谦　赵　欣　赵亚力　郑　青　郑艳华　朱江嵩

朱瑛培

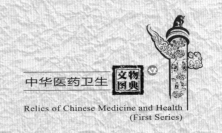

中华医药卫生 文物图典

Relics of Chinese Medicine and Health
(First Series)

本册编撰委员会

主　编　李经纬　梁　峻　刘学春

副主编　廖　果　吴鸿洲　康兴军　和中浚　刘小斌　杨金生

　　　　郑怀林　徐江雁　白建疆　黄　煌

编　委　李洪晓　梁永宣　王强虎　董树平　马　健　王　霞

　　　　张雅宗　朱德明　包哈申　张建青　郑　蓉　庄乾竹

　　　　李宏红　刘哲峰　王宏才　陈润东

总主译　白永权

主　译　吉　乐

副主译　詹菊红

译　者　王慧敏　迟征宇　张梦原　高　琛　王　媛　席　慧

　　　　牛笑语　吴耀均　黄　鋆　杨姣姣　蒋新蕾　姜雨孜

　　　　张　阳　姚　晔　郭　宁　刘雅恬

丛书策划委员会

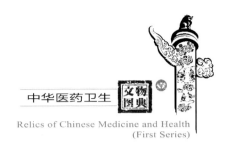

中华医药卫生 文物图典

Relics of Chinese Medicine and Health
(First Series)

序 言

　　探索天、地、人运动变化规律以及"气化物生"过程的相互关系，是人类永恒的课题。宇宙不可逆，地球不可逆，人生不可逆业已成为共识。天地造化形成自然，人类活动构成文化。文物既是文化的载体，又是物化的历史，还是文明的见证。

　　追求健康长寿是人类共同的夙愿。中华民族之所以繁衍昌盛，健康文化起了巨大的推动作用。由于古人谋求生存发展、应对环境变化产生的智慧，大多反映在以医药卫生为核心的健康文化之中，所以，习总书记说："中医药学是中国古代科学的瑰宝，也是打开中华文明宝库的钥匙"。

　　秉持文化大发展、大繁荣理念，中国中医科学院李经纬、梁峻等为负责人的科研团队在完成科技部"国家重点医药卫生文物收集调研和保护"课题获 2005 年度中华中医药学会科技二等奖基础上，又资鉴"夏商周断代工程""中华文明探源工程"等相关考古成果，用有重要价值的新出土文物置换原拍摄质量较差的文物，适当补充民族医药文物，共精选收载 5000 余件。经西安交通大学出版社申报，《中华医药卫生文物图典（一）》（以下简称《图典》）于 2013 年获得了国家出版基金的资助，并经专业翻译团队翻译，使《图典》得以面世。

　　文物承载的信息多元丰富，发掘解读其中蕴藏的智慧并非易事。 医药卫生文物更具有特殊性，除文物的一般属性外，还承载着传统医学发展史迹与促进健康的信息。运用历史唯物主义观察发掘文物信息，善于从生活文物中领悟卫生信息，才能准确解读其功能，也才能诠释其在民生健康中的历史作用，收到以古鉴今之效果。"历史是现实的根源"，任何一个民族都不能割断历史，史料都包含在文化中。"文化是民族的血脉，是人民的精神家园"，文化繁荣才能实现中华民族的伟大复兴。值本《图典》付梓之际，用"梳理文化之脉，必获健康之果"作为序言并和作者、读者共勉！

中央文史研究馆馆员

中国工程院院士　　王永炎

丁酉年仲夏

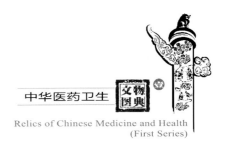

中华医药卫生 文物图典

Relics of Chinese Medicine and Health
(First Series)

前 言

　　文化是相对自然的概念，是考古界常用词汇。文物是文化的重要组成部分，既是文明的物证，又是物化的历史。狭义医药卫生文物是疾病防治模式语境下的解读，而广义医药卫生文物则是躯体、心态、环境适应三维健康模式下的诠释。中华民族是56个民族组成的多元一体大家庭，中华医药卫生文物当然包括各民族的健康文化遗存。

　　天地造化如造山、板块漂移、气候变迁、生物起源进化等形成自然。气化物生莫贵于人，即整个生物进化的最高成果是人类自身。广义而言，人类生存思维留下的痕迹即物质财富和精神财富总和构成文化，其一般的物化形式是视觉感知的文物、文献、胜迹等。其中质变标志明晰的文化如文字、文物、城市、礼仪等可称作文明。从唯物史观视角观察，狭义文化即精神财富，尤其体现人类精、气、神状态的事项，其本质也具有特殊物质属性，如量子也具有波粒二相性，这种粒子也是物质，无非运动方式特殊而已。现代所谓可重复验证的"科学"，事实上也是从文化中分离出来的事项，因此也是一种特殊文化形式。追求健康长寿是人类共同的夙愿。中华民族之所以繁衍昌盛，是因为健康文化异彩纷呈。中华优秀传统医药文化之所以博大精深，是因为其原创思维博大、格物致知精深，所以，习总书记说："中医药学是中国古代科学的瑰宝，也是打开中华文明宝库的钥匙"。

文化既反映时代、地域、民族分布、生产资料来源、技术水平等信息，又反映人类认知水平和生存智慧。发掘解读文物、文献中蕴藏的健康知识和灵动智慧，首先是从事健康工作者的责任和义务。《易经》设有"观"卦，人类作为观察者，不仅要积极收藏展陈文物，而且要善于捕捉文物倾诉的信息，汲取养分，启迪思维，收到古为今用之效果。墨子三表法，首先一表即"本之于古者圣王之事"，也是强调古代史实的重要性。"历史是现实的根源"，现实是未来的基础。任何一个国家、地区、民族都不能割断历史、忽略基础，这个基础就是文化。"文化是民族的血脉，是人民的精神家园"。文化繁荣才能驱动各项事业发展，才能实现中华民族的伟大复兴。

人类从类人猿分化出来。"禄丰古猿禄丰种"是云南禄丰发现的类人猿化石，距今七八百万年。距今 200 万年前人类进入旧石器时代，直立行走，打制石器产生工具意识，管理火种，是所谓"燧人氏"时代。中国留存有更新世早、中期的元谋、蓝田、北京人等遗址。距今 10 万—5 万年前，人类进入旧石器时代中期，即早期智人阶段，脑容量增加，和欧洲、非洲人种相比，原始蒙古人种颧骨前突等，是所谓"伏羲氏"时代。中国发现的马坝、长阳、丁村人等较典型。距今 5 万—1 万年前，人类进入旧石器时代晚期，即晚期智人阶段，细石器、骨角器等遍布全国，山顶洞、柳江、资阳人等较典型。

中石器时代距今约 1 万年，是旧石器时代向新石器时代的短暂过渡期，弓箭发明，狗被驯化。河南灵井、陕西沙苑遗址等作为代表。距今 1 万—公元前 2600 年前后，人类进入新石器时代，磨光石器、烧制陶器，出现农业村落并饲养家畜，是所谓"神农氏"时代。公元前 7000 年以来，在甲、骨、陶、石等载体上出现契刻符号、七音阶骨笛乐器等，反映出人文气息趋浓。公元前 6000—公元前 3500 年的老官台、裴李岗、河姆渡、马家浜、仰韶等文化遗址，彰显出先民围绕生存健康问题所做的各种努力。

公元前 4800 年以来，以关中、晋南、豫西为中心形成的仰韶文化，是中原史前文化的重要标志。以半坡、庙底沟类型为典型，自公元前 3500 年走向繁荣，属于锄耕粟黍稻兼营渔猎饲养猪鸡经济方式，彩陶尤其发达。公元前 4400—公元前 3300 年，长江中游的大溪文化，薄胎彩陶和白陶发达。公元前 4300—公元前 2500 年山东丰岛的大汶口文化，红陶为主。公元前 3500 年前后，辽东的红山文化原始宗教发展。公元前 3300 年以来，长江下游由河姆渡、马家浜文化衍续的良渚文化和陇西的马家窑文化、江淮间的薛家岗文化时趋发达。

公元前 2600—公元前 2000 年，黄河中下游龙山文化群形成，冶铸铜器，制作玉器，土坯、石灰、夯筑技术开始应用。公元前 2697 年，轩辕战败炎帝（有说其后裔）、蚩尤而为黄帝纪元元年。黄帝西巡访贤，"至岐见岐伯，引载而归，访于治道"。其引归地"溱洧襟带于前，梅泰环拱于后"，即今河南新密市古城寨。岐黄答问，构建《黄帝内经》健康知识体系，中华文明从关注民生健康起步。颛顼改革宗教，神职人员出现；帝喾修身节用，帝尧和合百国，舜同律度量衡，大禹疏导治水，中华民族不断繁衍昌盛。

公元前 2070 年，禹之子启以豫西晋南为中心建立夏王朝，二里头青铜文化为其特征，半地穴、窑洞、地面建筑并存。饮食卫生器具、酒器增多。朱砂安神作用在宫殿应用。公元前 1600 年，商灭夏。偃师商城设有铸铜作坊。公元前 1300 年，盘庚迁殷，使用甲骨文。武丁时期青铜浑铸、分铸并存。公元前 1056 年，相传周"文王被殷纣拘于羑里，演《周易》，成六十四卦"。公元前 1046 年，武王克商建周，定都镐京。青铜器始铸长篇铭文，周原发掘出微型甲骨文字。公元前 770 年，平王东迁。虢国铸铜柄铁剑。公元前 753 年，秦国设置史官。公元前 707 年出现蝗灾、公元前 613 年出现"哈雷彗星"，均被孔子载入《春秋》。公元前 221 年，秦始皇统一中国，多元一体民族大家庭形成，中华医药卫生文物异彩纷呈。

中国是治史大国，历来重视发展文化博物事业，1955 年成立卫生部中医研究院时就设置医史研究室，1982 年中国医史文献研究所成立时复建中国医史博物馆研究收藏展陈文物。2000—2003 年，经王永炎院士、姚乃礼院长等呼吁，科技部批准立项，由李经纬、梁峻为负责人的团队完成"国家重点医药卫生文物收集调研和保护"项目任务，受到科技部项目验收组专家的高度评价，获中华中医药学会科技进步二等奖。2013 年，在国家出版基金资助下，课题组对部分文物重新拍摄或必要置换、充实民族医药文物后，由西安交通大学出版社编辑、组聘国内一流翻译团队英译说明文字付梓，受到国家中医药博物馆筹备工作领导小组和办公室的高度重视。

"物以类聚"，《图典》主要依据文物质地、种类分为 9 卷，计有陶瓷，金属，纸质，竹木，玉石、织品及标本，壁画石刻及遗址，少数民族文物，其他，备考等卷。同卷下主要根据历史年代或小类分册设章。每卷下的历史时段不求统一。遵循上述规则将《图典》划分为21册，总计收载文物5000余件。对每件文物的描述，除质地、规格、馆藏等基本要素外，重点描述其在民生健康中的作用。对少数暂不明确的事项在括号中注明待考。对引自各博物馆的材料除在文物后列出馆藏外，还在书后再次统一列出馆名或参考书目，以充分尊重其馆藏权，也同时维护本典作者的引用权。

21世纪，围绕人类健康的生命科学将飞速发展，但科学离不开文化，文化离不开文物。发掘文物承载的信息为现实服务，谨引用横渠先生四言之两语："为天地立心，为生民立命"，既作为编撰本《图典》之宗旨，也是我们践行国家"一带一路"倡议的具体努力。希冀通过本《图典》的出版发行，教育国人，提振中华民族精神；走向世界，为人类健康事业贡献力量。

李经纬　梁峻　刘学春

2017年6月于北京

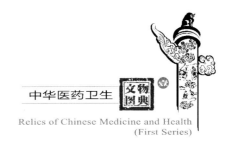

中华医药卫生文物图典

Relics of Chinese Medicine and Health
(First Series)

目 录

第一章 清（1840 年以前）

串铃 ……………………………………002

串铃 ……………………………………004

铜串铃 …………………………………006

铜串铃 …………………………………008

圆铁铃 …………………………………010

铜药臼 …………………………………011

铁药臼 …………………………………012

铁药臼 …………………………………013

铜药臼 …………………………………014

铜药臼 …………………………………016

药锤 ……………………………………017

铜药臼 …………………………………018

太医院药臼、杵 ………………………019

御生堂药臼、药杵 ……………………020

药臼 ……………………………………022

御生堂金锅铜铲 ………………………024

臼 ………………………………………026

带杵药臼 ………………………………028

药臼 ……………………………………030

带杵药臼 ………………………………032

铜药臼 …………………………………034

铁药碾槽 ………………………………036

小碾槽 …………………………………037

太医院药碾 ……………………………038

铜碾药船 ………………………………039

碾药船 …………………………………040

小铁刀 …………………………………042

小铁刀 …………………………………043

铁药刀 …………………………………044

铜切药刀 ………………………………046

铁药钳 …………………………………047

铁锻药钳 ………………………………048

太医院药锅 ……………………………049

太医院双耳药筛 ………………………050

太医院盖碗药筛 ………………………052

御药房温药壶 …………………………054

御生堂药酒壶 …………………………056

铜药匙 …………………………………058

铜药勺头 ………………………………060

勺 ………………………………………062

匙 ………………………………………063

匕 ………………………………………064

铜半圆药瓶 ……………………………065

链环药瓶 ………………………………066

长颈扁药瓶 ……………………………069

铜药瓶 …………………………………070

铜扁药瓶 ………………………………072

麝香银盒 ………………………………074

药盒 ……………………………………076

药盒 ……………………………………078

铜药盒 080

御生堂针具 082

外科手术器械 084

中医外科器械 087

外科器具 088

中医外科用具 090

手术器具 091

中医外科器械 093

铁质小针、刀、铜匙 094

外科斜刃刀 096

外科斜刃刀 098

外科斜刃刀 100

外科斜刃刀 102

外科斜刃刀 104

外科斜刃刀 106

外科斜刃刀 108

外科斜刃刀 110

外科斜刃刀 112

外科斜刃刀 114

外科斜刃刀 116

外科斜刃刀 118

外科斜刃刀 120

柳叶刀 122

外科弯刃刀 124

外科弯刃刀 126

外科弯刃刀 128

外科弯刃刀 130

外科弯刃刀 132

外科弯刃刀 134

外科弯刃刀 136

外科圆刃铲刀 138

外科圆刃铲刀 140

外科圆刃铲刀 142

外科圆刃铲刀 144

外科尖刀 146

外科尖刀 148

外科钩镰刀 150

外科钩镰刀 152

外科钩镰刀 154

外科钩镰刀 156

外科两用器 158

外科簇尖刺锥 160

外科簇尖刺锥 162

外科簇尖刺锥 164

外科簇尖刺锥 166

外科簇尖刺锥 168

外科簇尖刺锥 170

外科簇尖刺锥 172

外科斜刃刀 174

外科簇尖刺锥 176

外科簇尖刺锥 178

外科簇尖刺锥 180

外科尖棱锥 182

外科尖棱锥 184

秤 186

铁刀 187

铜铲 188

锡罐 190

铜壶 192

铝参壶 194

双桃锡酒壶 197

温酒器 198

铝茶壶 200

铜杯 202

铜酒杯 203

铜箸 204

小铜勺 206

铁像 207

铜像 208

铜盆 209

铜刻花匜 211

铜盆 212

盆 214

盆 216

铁盆 218

圆铁盒 220

圆铁盒 222
铁盒 224
银帕架 226
铜镜 227
铜镜 228
百子图镜 231
嘉庆慎思堂十二生肖柄镜 233
铜发钗 234
清宫御用鎏金耳挖勺 235
金嵌珠翠耳挖勺簪 237
铜二须 238
银三须 239
银三须 240
银三须 242
银五须 244
清理耳鼻工具 246
清理耳鼻工具 248
剃刀 250
指甲套 252
指甲套 254
铜手炉 256
八角铜手炉 258
佛手 259
熏炉 260
熏炉 262
熏炉 264
熏炉 266
炼丹炉 268
蹴鞠图漆绘铜牌 271
手柄铜斧 272
铁云牌 274
铁磬 276
铁灯 278
油灯盏 280
铁灯 282
油灯盏座 284
铜灯 286
铜油灯 289

铝台灯 290
铜灭蚊灯 292
铜鼻烟壶 294
画珐琅人物纹烟壶 296
水烟筒 299
烟枪头 301
小铜鸽子像 302
铜币 304

第二章　近现代

许浚像 306
铜印（复制） 308
焦易堂半身铜像 310
傅连暲墨盒 312
陆坤豪挂号牌 314
陆坤豪挂号牌 316
中华医学会徽章 318
中央国医馆徽章 320
上海中医专科学校证章 322
北京协和医院建院纪念章 324
"女子产科学校"印章 327
上海牙医师公会铜印 328
上海牙医师公会铜印 330
杵臼 332
臼 334
铜药臼 337
药臼 338
小铁药碾 340
药碾船 341
铁碾槽 342
刀 343
铁药刀 344
铜药匙 346
铜药勺 347
铜药勺 348
铜药勺 349
药罐 350

药盒 ……………………… 351
药盒 ……………………… 352
药盒 ……………………… 354
药盒 ……………………… 356
药盒 ……………………… 358
药盒 ……………………… 360
药盒 ……………………… 362
药盒 ……………………… 364
药盒 ……………………… 366
药盒 ……………………… 368
药盒 ……………………… 370
药盒 ……………………… 372
药盒 ……………………… 374
药瓶 ……………………… 376
熬药罐 …………………… 378
"午时茶" 模具 …………… 380
鼻箔管 …………………… 382
药鼓 ……………………… 384
药鼓 ……………………… 386
药鼓 ……………………… 388
喷药粉器 ………………… 390
喷药粉器 ………………… 392
药鼓 ……………………… 394
铜膏药刀 ………………… 395
刀 ………………………… 396
刀 ………………………… 397
刀 ………………………… 398
刀 ………………………… 399
银九针 …………………… 400
针 ………………………… 402
针 ………………………… 403
针 ………………………… 404
镊子 ……………………… 405
剪 ………………………… 406
针筒 ……………………… 407
"太乙神针" 铜藏针筒 …… 408
针灸铜人 ………………… 410
拔火罐 …………………… 412

温灸器 …………………… 414
灸条夹 …………………… 415
佩饰 ……………………… 416
佩饰 ……………………… 417
锡罐 ……………………… 418
锡火锅 …………………… 420
铜酒杯 …………………… 421
小锡壶 …………………… 422
匙 ………………………… 424
匙 ………………………… 425
匙 ………………………… 426
匙 ………………………… 427
勺 ………………………… 428
匙 ………………………… 429
铜勺 ……………………… 430
铜马勺 …………………… 431
洗 ………………………… 432
铜叉 ……………………… 434
唾盂 ……………………… 437
唾盂 ……………………… 438
唾盂 ……………………… 440
景泰蓝小蓝瓶 …………… 442
灭蚊灯 …………………… 444
铜铃 ……………………… 446
铜铃（甩子） …………… 447
铁钟 ……………………… 448
铜镰 ……………………… 450
铜镰 ……………………… 451
铜镰 ……………………… 452
酒瓶 ……………………… 453
铜水烟袋 ………………… 455
烟嘴 ……………………… 456
旱烟管 …………………… 458
铜烟袋锅 ………………… 460
铜烟灯 …………………… 461

索引 …………………… 462
参考文献 ……………… 473

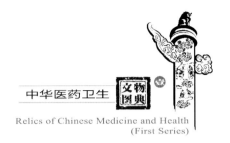

中华医药卫生
Relics of Chinese Medicine and Health
(First Series)

Contents

Chapter One   Qing Dynasty (Before 1840)

Ring-like Bell 002

Ring-like Bell 004

Copper Ring-like Bell 006

Copper Ring-like Bell 008

Round Iron Bell 010

Copper Medicine Mortar 011

Iron Medicine Mortar 012

Iron Medicine Mortar 013

Copper Medicine Mortar 014

Copper Medicine Mortar 016

Medicine Hammer 017

Copper Medicine Mortar 018

Medicine Mortar and Pestle of Imperial Hospital 019

Medicine Mortar with Pestle of Yu Sheng Tang Drugstore 020

Medicine Mortar 022

Gold Pot and Bronze Shovel of Yu Sheng Tang Drugstore 024

Mortar 026

Medicine Mortar with Pestle 028

Medicine Mortar 030

Medicine Mortar with Pestle 032

Copper Medicine Mortar 034

Iron Medicine Mill Groove 036

Small Mill Groove 037

Medicine Mill of Imperial Hospital 038

Ship-like Copper Medicine Mill 039

Ship-like Medicine Mill 040

Small Iron Knife 042

Small Iron Knife 043

Iron Medical Knife 044

Copper Knife for Slicing Medicine 046

Iron Medicine Tong 047

Iron-forged Medicine Tong 048

Medicine Cauldron of Imperial Hospital 049

Two-Handle Medicine Sieve of Imperial Hospital 050

Medicine Sieve Bowl with Cover of Imperial Hospital..........052

Medicine Heating Pot of Imperial Pharmacy.......054

Medical Wine Pot of Yu Sheng Tang 056

Copper Medicine Spoon 058

Head of Copper Medicine Spoon........................060

Spoon 062

Spoon 063

An Ancient Type of Spoon 064

Copper Semicircular Medicine Bottle 065

Medicine Bottles Connected with Hinges............066

Flattened Medicine Bottle with a Long Neck 069

Coppery Medicine Bottle 070

Copper Flattened Medicine Bottle 072

Silver Box for Musk 074

Medicine Box 076

Medicine Box..078

Copper Medicine Box 080

Acupuncture Needles from Yu Sheng Tang Drugstore 082

Surgical Instruments 084

Traditional Chinese Surgical Instruments 087

Surgical Instruments 088

Traditional Chinese Surgical Instruments 090

Surgical Instruments 091

Traditional Chinese Surgical Instruments 093

Iron Needles, Knife and Copper Spoon 094

Surgical Scalpel with Oblique Blade 096

Surgical Scalpel with Oblique Blade 098

Surgical Scalpel with Oblique Blade 100

Surgical Scalpel with Oblique Blade 102

Surgical Scalpel with Oblique Blade 104

Surgical Scalpel with Oblique Blade 106

Surgical Scalpel with Oblique Blade 108

Surgical Scalpel with Oblique Blade 110

Surgical Scalpel with Oblique Blade 112

Surgical Scalpel with Oblique Blade 114

Surgical Scalpel with Oblique Blade 116

Surgical Scalpel with Oblique Blade 118

Surgical Scalpel with Oblique Edge 120

Lancet (Liu Ye Dao) 122

Surgical Knife with Curving Edge 124

Surgical Knife with Curving Edge 126

Surgical Knife with Curving Edge 128

Surgical Knife with Curving Edge 130

Surgical Knife with Curving Edge 132

Surgical Knife with Curving Edge 134

Surgical Knife with Curving Edge 136

Surgical Scraper Knife with Round Edge 138

Surgical Scraper Knife with Round Edge 140

Surgical Scraper Knife with Round Edge 142

Surgical Scraper Knife with Round Edge 144

Surgical Sharp Knife 146

Surgical Sharp Knife 148

Surgical Sickle-like Knife with Hook 150

Surgical Sickle-like Knife with Hook 152

Surgical Sickle-like Knife with Hook 154

Surgical Sickle-like Knife with Hook 156

Surgical Appliance of Two-Purpose 158

Surgical Awl with Pointed Tip 160

Surgical Awl with Pointed Tip 162

Surgical Awl with Pointed Tip 164

Surgical Awl with Pointed Tip 166

Surgical Awl with Pointed Tip 168

Surgical Awl with Pointed Tip 170

Surgical Awl with Pointed Tip 172

Surgical Knife with Oblique Edge 174

Surgical Awl with Pointed Tip 176

Surgical Awl with Pointed Tip 178

Surgical Awl with Pointed Tip 180

Surgical Awl with Sharp and Pyramid-Shaped Tip.................182

Surgical Awl with Sharp and Pyramid-Shaped Tip.................184

Scale...186

Iron Knife..187

Copper Shovel...188

Tin Can..190

Copper Pot...192

Aluminum Pot for Cooking Ginseng Soup...........................194

Tin Flagon in the Shape of Two Peaches 197

Utensil for Heating Wine 198

Aluminum Tea Pot 200

Copper Cup...202

Copper Wine Cup...203

Copper Chopsticks..204

Small Copper Spoon..206

Iron Statue..207

Copper Statue..208

Copper Basin...209

Copper Gourd-shaped Ladle with Engraved Designs............211

Copper Basin...212

Basin 214

Basin 216

Iron Basin..218

Round Iron Container 220

Round Iron Container 222

Iron Container 224

Silver Handkerchief Holder 226

Copper Mirror 227

Copper Mirror 228

Mirror with Children Patterns 231

Mirror of Severance Hall Made in Jiaqing Periods,

with Chinese Zodiac Patterns 233

Copper Hairpin 234

Imperial Gilding Ear Pick 235

Gold Ear-picker Hairpin Inlaid with Pearl and Jadeite 237

Copper Whisker-like Tools of Two Pieces 238

Silver Whisker-like Tools of Three Pieces 239

Silver Whisker-like Tools of Three Pieces 240

Silver Whisker-like Tools of Three Pieces 242

Silver Whisker-like Tools of Five Pieces 244

A Nose and Ear Cleaning Tool 246

A Nose and Ear Cleaning Tool 248

Shaver 250

Fingernail Cover 252

Fingernail Cover 254

Copper Handwarmer 256

Octagon Copper Handwarmer 258

Censer in the Shape of Fingered Citron 259

Censer 260

Censer 262

Censer 264

Censer 266

Alchemy Furnace 268

Lacquered Bronze Plate with Cuju Painting 271

Copper Axe with Handle 272

Iron "Yun-pai" 274

Iron "Qing" 276

Iron Lamp 278

Oil Lamp 280

Iron Lamp 282

Oil Lamp Pedestal 284

Copper Lamp 286

Copper Oil Lamp 289

Aluminum Table Lamp 290

Copper Mosquito-Killing Lamp 292

Copper Snuff Bottle 294

Snuff Bottle with Enamel Figure Painting 296

Chinese Water Pipe 299

Smoking Pipe Head 301

Small Copper Pigeon 302

Copper Coin 304

Chapter Two   Modern Times

Statue of Xu Jun 306

Copper Seal (Copy) 308

Half-Length Copper Statue of Jiao Yitang 310

Fu Lianzhang's Ink Box 312

Registration Tablet of Lu Kunhao 314

Registration Tablet of Lu Kunhao 316

Badges of the Chinese Medical Association 318

Badges of the Central State Hospital 320

Badge of Shanghai Traditional Chinese Medicine

Specialized School 322

Establishment Souvenir Badge of the Peking Union

Medical College Hospital 324

Seal of the Female Obstetrics School 327

Copper Seal of Shanghai Dentist Association 328

Copper Seal of Shanghai Dental Association 330

Mortar with Pestle 332

Mortar 334

Copper Medicinal Mortar 337

Medicinal Mortar 338

Small Iron Medicinal Crusher 340

Ship-like Medicinal Crusher 341

Iron Mill Groove 342

Knife 343

Iron Medicinal Knife 344

Copper Medicinal Spoon 346

Copper Medicinal Ladle 347

Copper Medicinal Ladle 348

Copper Medicinal Ladle 349

Gallipot 350

Medicine Box 351

Medicine Box 352

Medicine Box 354

Medicine Box 356

Medicine Box 358

Medicine Box 360

Medicine Box 362

Medicine Box 364

Medicine Box 366

Medicine Box 368

Medicine Box 370

Medicine Box 372

Medicine Box 374

Medicine Bottles 376

The Pot for Decocting Herbal Medicine 378

"Wu Shi Cha" (Herbal Tea) Mould 380

Nasal Tube Covered with Foil 382

Drum-like Medical Instrument 384

Drum-like Medical Instrument 386

Drum-like Medical Instrument 388

Medical Spray Tube 390

Medical Spray Tube 392

Drum-like Medical Instrument 394

Copper Medical Plaster Knife 395

Knife 396

Knife 397

Knife 398

Knife 399

Silver "Nine Needles" 400

Needle 402

Needle 403

Needle 404

Tweezers 405

Scissors 406

Syringe 407

Copper Cylinder of "Taiyi Miraculous Needles" 408

Copper Acupuncture Status 410

Cupping Glass 412

Moxa Burner 414

Clamp for Moxa Stick 415

Accessory 416

Accessory 417

Tin Pot 418

Tin Stove 420

Copper Wine Cup 421

Small Tin Pot 422

Spoon 424

Spoon 425

Spoon 426

Spoon 427

Spoon 428

Spoon 429

Copper Spoon 430

Copper Ladle 431

Washer 432

Copper Fork 434

Spittoon 437

Spittoon 438

Spittoon 440

Small Cloisonne Vase 442

Mosquito Killer Lamp 444

Copper Bell 446

Copper Bell (Hollow Swage) 447

Iron Bell 448

Copper Sickle 450

Copper Sickle 451

Copper Sickle 452

Wine Bottle 453

Copper Hookah 455

Tobacco Pipe 456

Tobacco Pipe 458

Copper Tobacco Pipe 460

Copper Tobacco Burner 461

Index 468

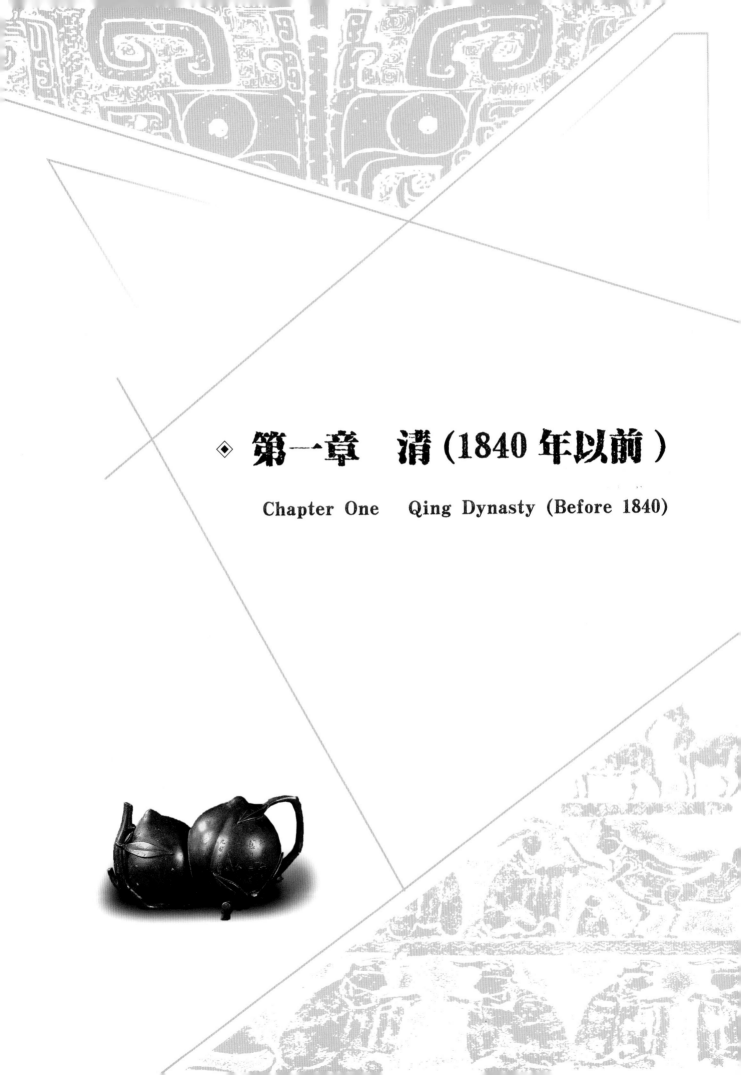

◇ 第一章 清（1840 年以前）

Chapter One Qing Dynasty (Before 1840)

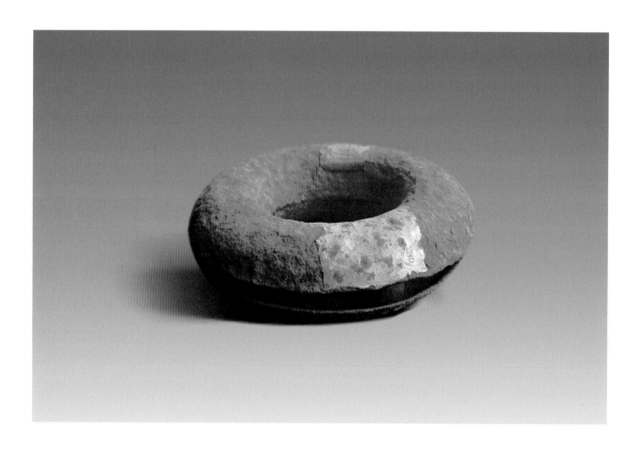

串铃

清

铁质

内径 4.5 厘米，外径 11.5 厘米

Ring-like Bell

Qing Dynasty

Iron

Inner Diameter 4.5 cm/ Outer Diameter 11.5 cm

空心铁环状，内置铁球，一摇即响。串铃，

也称"虎撑"或"虎衔"，外出行医用具。

江苏省中医药博物馆藏

This is a hollow tubular iron ring with an iron
ball inside which rings while being shaken. The
ring-like bell, also called as "Hu Cheng" or "Hu
Xian" (legend has it that Sun Simiao once put it
inside a tiger's mouth to protect himself when
he pulled out the bone stuck in its throat), was a
tool carried by doctors who went out to practice
medicine.

Preserved in Jiangsu Museum of Traditional
Chinese Medicine

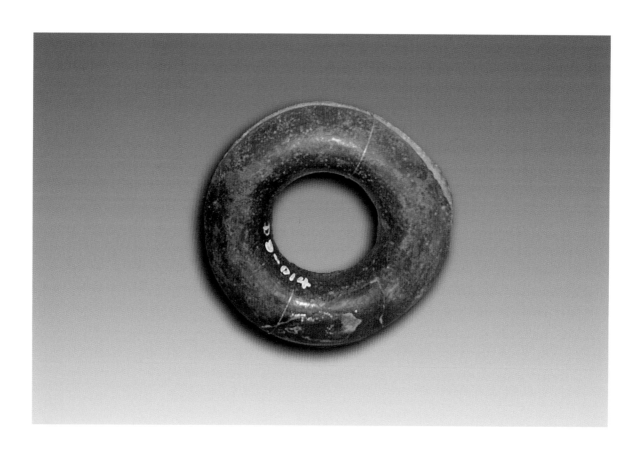

串铃

清

铁质

直径 11.2 厘米，重 400 克

Ring-like Bell

Qing Dynasty

Iron

Diameter 11.2 cm/ Weight 400 g

圆形中间有一孔，完整无损。医疗器具。山西省临猗地区征集。

陕西医史博物馆藏

There is a hole in the middle of the round bell which is in good shape. It was used as a medical instrument and was collected from Linqi region, Shanxi Province.

Preserved in Shaanxi Museum of Medical History

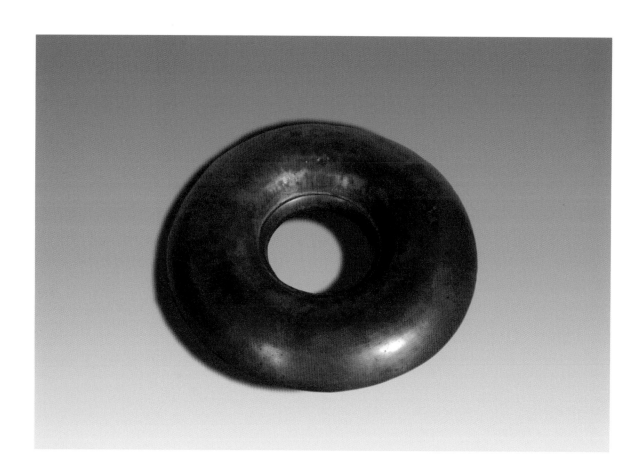

铜串铃

清

铜质

外径 12.6 厘米，内径 4 厘米，高 3.4 厘米

Copper Ring-like Bell

Qing Dynasty

Copper

Outer Diameter 12.6 cm/ Inner Diameter 4 cm/ Height 3.4 cm

环状，该藏表面光滑，环状空心，环外缘有一圈窄缝隙便于声音产生，环内有两个金属串珠，是走方医行医用具。1954 年入藏。保存基本完好。

中华医学会 / 上海中医药大学医史博物馆藏

The hollow ring-like bell has a circular smooth surface, with a narrow slit for sound production on the outer layer and two medal beads inside. It was used as a medical appliance. The bell, collected in 1954, is still in good condition. Preserved in Chinese Medical Association/ Museum of Chinese Medicine, Shanghai University of Traditional Chinese Medicine

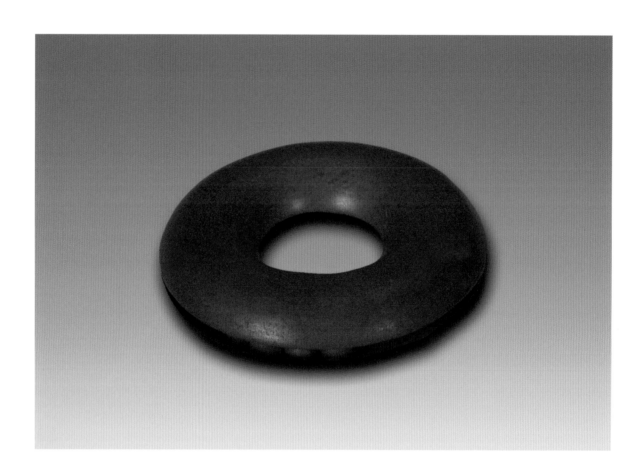

铜串铃

清

铜质

外径 13.3 厘米，内径 4.9 厘米，高 3.4 厘米

Copper Ring-like Bell

Qing Dynasty

Copper

Outer Diameter 13.3 cm/ Inner Diameter 4.9 cm/ Height 3.4 cm

该藏表面光滑，环状空心，环外缘有一圈窄缝隙便于声音产生，环内有两颗金属串珠，是走方医行医用具。1959 年入藏。保存基本完好。

中华医学会 / 上海中医药大学医史博物馆藏

The hollow ring-like bell has a circular smooth surface, with a narrow slit for sound production on the outer layer and two medal beads inside. It was used as a medical appliance for a wandering doctor. The bell, collected in 1959, is still in good condition.

Preserved in Chinese Medical Association/ Museum of Chinese Medicine, Shanghai University of Traditional Chinese Medicine

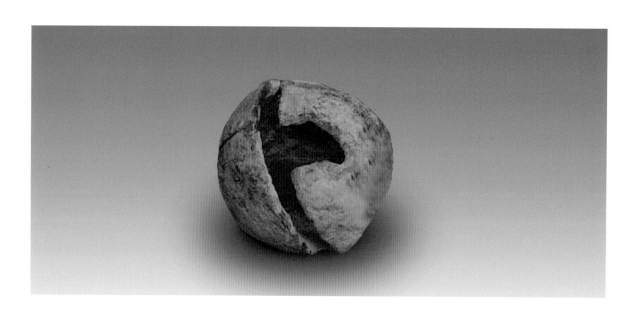

圆铁铃

清

铁质

直径 4 厘米，重 100 克

圆球状。车饰部件。有残损。

陕西医史博物馆藏

Round Iron Bell

Qing Dynasty

Iron

Diameter 4 cm/ Weight 100 g

This bell, damaged and ball-shaped, is a decorative component for carriage.

Preserved in Shaanxi Museum of Medical History

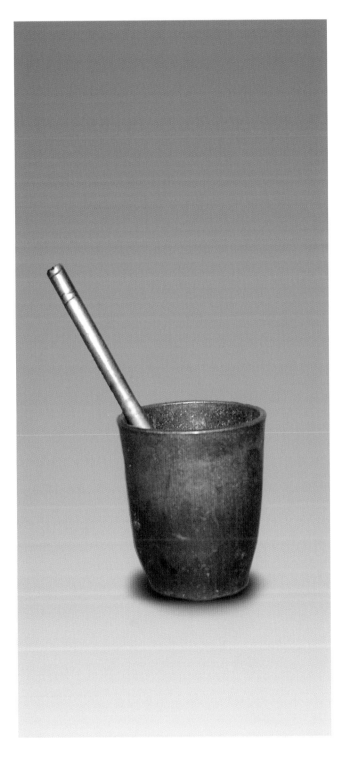

铜药臼

清

铜质

口径9.2厘米，底径6厘米，通高10.4厘米，
重1300克

敞口，直腹，平底，带一铜杵。捣药器具。
完整无损。

陕西医史博物馆藏

Copper Medicine Mortar

Qing Dynasty

Copper

Mouth Diameter 9.2 cm/ Bottom Diameter 6 cm/
Height 10.4 cm/ Weight 1,300 g

The mortar has an open mouth, an upright
belly, a flat bottom and a copper pestle. It was
used for pounding medicine and is still in good
shape now.

Preserved in Shaanxi Museum of Medical History

铁药臼

清

铁质

口径 12.5 厘米，底径 12 厘米，通高 13 厘米，重 4500 克

直口，圆腹，直底座，下底座有"川"字纹，带杵。捣药器具。有修补。

陕西医史博物馆藏

Iron Medicine Mortar

Qing Dynasty

Iron

Mouth Diameter 12.5 cm/ Bottom Diameter 12 cm/ Height 13 cm/ Weight 4,500 g

The mortar has an upright mouth, a round belly and an upright pedestal and a pestle. Patterns like Chinese character " 川 "(Chuan) are on the lower pedestal. It was used for pounding medicine and has been repaired.

Preserved in Shaanxi Museum of Medical History

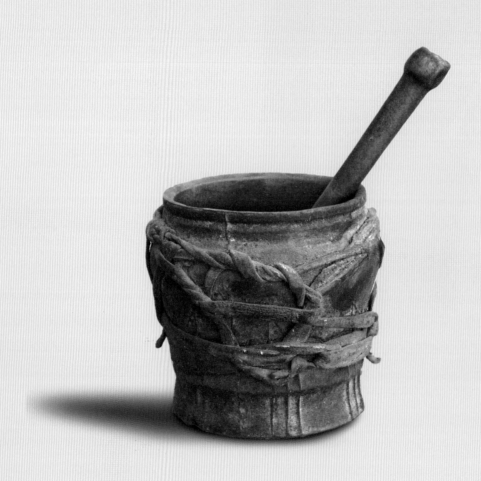

铁药臼

清

铁质

口径 10.4 厘米，底径 19.8 厘米，通高 20 厘米，重 5400 克

侈口，折肩，五蹼足。完整无损。制药器具。陕西省澄城县善化乡征集。

陕西医史博物馆藏

Iron Medicine Mortar

Qing Dynasty

Iron

Mouth Diameter 10.4 cm/ Bottom Diameter 19.8 cm/ Height 20 cm/ Weight 5,400 g

The mortar has a large mouth, bended shoulders and five webfeet. It was used as a pharmaceutical appliance and is well-preserved. The relic was collected from Shanhua Village, Chengcheng County, Shaanxi Province.

Preserved in Shaanxi Museum of Medical History

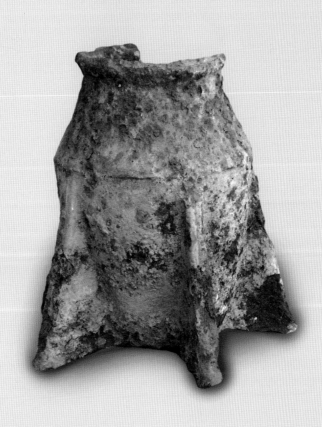

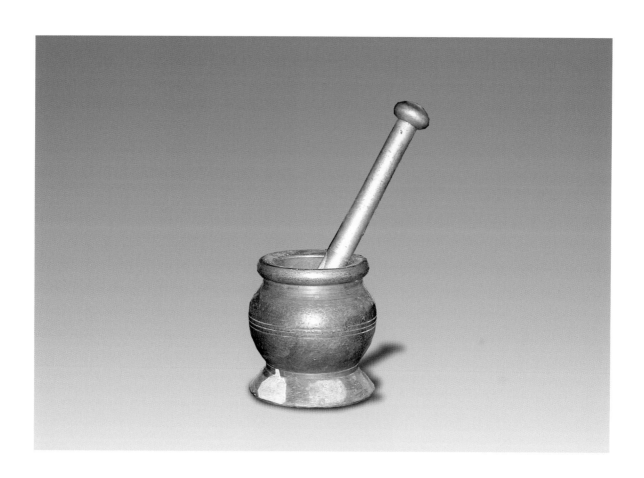

铜药臼

清

铜质

口径 9.5 厘米，底径 11 厘米，通高 11.5 厘米，重 5000 克

Copper Medicine Mortar

Qing Dynasty

Copper

Mouth Diameter 9.5 cm/ Bottom Diameter 11 cm/ Height 11.5 cm/ Weight 5,000 g

平口沿，鼓腹，倒喇叭座，腹有两道弦纹，

带一铜杆。捣药器具。完整无损。

陕西医史博物馆藏

The mortar has a flat mouth edge, a swelling

belly, which is decorated with two circles of

string pattern, an inverted trumpet-like bottom

and a copper pestle. It was used for pounding

medicine and is still in good shape now.

Preserved in Shaanxi Museum of Medical History

铜药臼

清

铜质

口径 9 厘米，底径 6 厘米，通高 22 厘米，重 1600 克

子母口，直斜腹，平底，带盖带一杵。捣药器具。完整无损。

陕西医史博物馆藏

Copper Medicine Mortar

Qing Dynasty

Copper

Mouth Diameter 9 cm/ Bottom Diameter 6 cm/ Height 22 cm/ Weight 1,600 g

The mortar has a pair of matching mouths, an upright and oblique belly, a flat bottom, a cover and a pestle. It was used for pounding medicine and is still in good shape now.

Preserved in Shaanxi Museum of Medical History

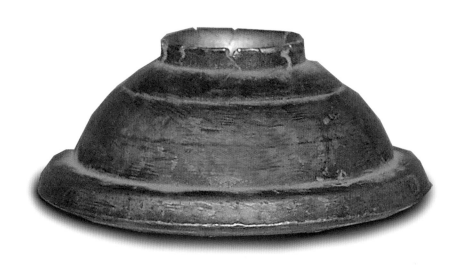

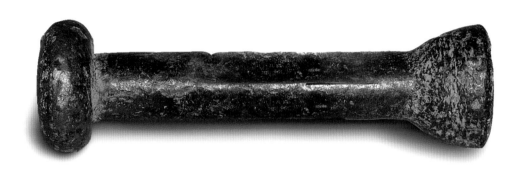

药锤

清

铜质

长 2.8 厘米，重 500 克

呈亚铃状。一端稍大呈椭圆形，一端半球形作捣物用，底面平整。医用器具。完整无损。

陕西医史博物馆藏

Medicine Hammer

Qing Dynasty

Copper

Length 2.8 cm/ Weight 500 g

This dumbbell-shaped medicine hammer has a larger oval-shaped end and a hemispheric end with flat bottom which is used for pounding medicine. It was used as a medical appliance and is still in good shape.

Preserved in Shaanxi Museum of Medical History

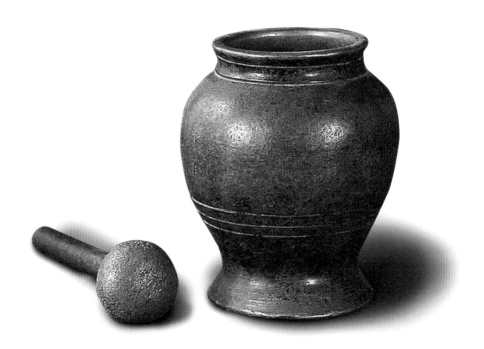

铜药臼

清

铜质

腹径 23 厘米，底径 6 厘米，高 15 厘米

侈口，束颈，鼓腹，底平外撇。颈与腹刻有弦纹，带杵。制药用具。

上海中医药博物馆藏

Copper Medicine Mortar

Qing Dynasty

Copper

Belly Diameter 23 cm/ Bottom Diameter 6 cm/ Height 15 cm

This is a mortar with a wide flared mouth, a converging neck, a bulging belly and a flat-out bottom. String patterns were carved on the neck and belly. The mortar with the pestle is used for mashing herbs.

Preserved in Shanghai Museum of Traditional Chinese Medicine

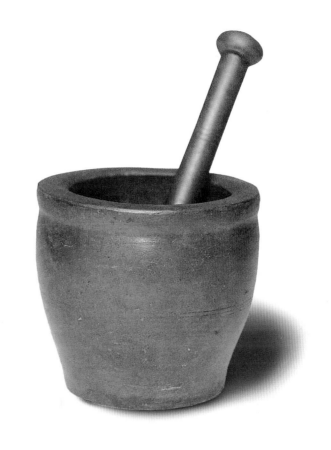

太医院药臼、杵

清

铜质

臼：腹径 19.5 厘米，底径 14 厘米，高 18 厘米

杵：长 31 厘米

罐形，表面光洁。捣药用的器具。

中国国家博物馆藏

Medicine Mortar and Pestle of Imperial Hospital

Qing Dynasty

Copper

Mortar: Belly Diameter 19.5 cm/ Bottom Diameter 14 cm/ Height 18 cm

Pestle: Length 31 cm

This mortar with smooth surface is used for mashing herbs.

Preserved in National Museum of China

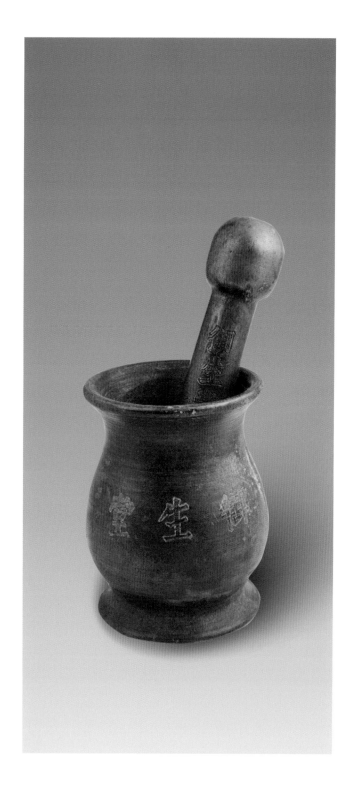

御生堂药臼、药杵

清

铜质

药臼：口径 14 厘米，高 26 厘米

杵：长 36 厘米，底径 6 厘米

Medicine Mortar with Pestle of Yu Sheng Tang Drugstore

Qing Dynasty

Bronze

Mortar: Mouth Diameter 14 cm/ Height 26 cm

Pestle: Length 36 cm/ Bottom Diameter 6 cm

侈口，束颈，鼓腹，腹上刻"御生堂"字样，

平底，圈足。带杵。用于捣碎药材。

北京御生堂中医药博物馆藏

This mortar has a flared mouth, a contracted
neck, a flat bottom, a ring foot and a bulged
belly with the inscriptions reading "Yu Sheng
Tang" on it. A pestle goes with it. It was used
for smashing medicinal materials.

Preserved in Chinese Medicine Museum of
Beijing Yu Sheng Tang Drugstore

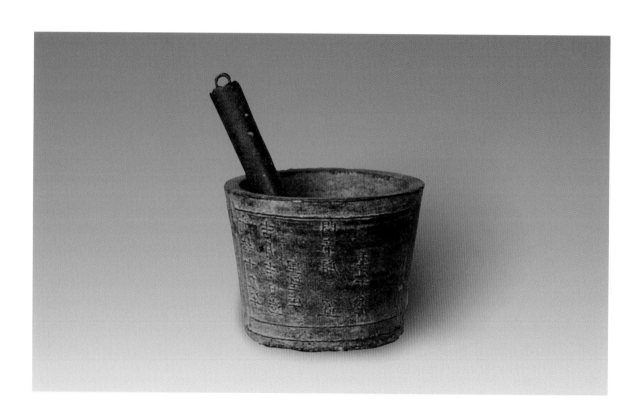

药臼

清

合金

药臼：口径 40 厘米，底径 32 厘米，高 36 厘米

杵：长 52 厘米

Medicine Mortar

Qing Dynasty

Alloy

Mortar: Mouth Diameter 40 cm/ Bottom Diameter 32 cm/ Height 36 cm

Pestle: Length 52 cm

敞口，平沿，斜腹，平底。臼体上有铭文"光绪十九年吉月吉日造里望庄关帝庙置重八十余斤"。带杵。关帝庙供人们捣药之用。

北京御生堂中医药博物馆藏

The mortar has a flared mouth, a contracted belly and a flat bottom. The inscriptions on its body suggest that it was made in the nineteenth year of Emperor Guangxu's Reign for the temple of Lord Guan and the weight is more than 40 kg. A pestle goes with it. It was used for pounding medicine.

Preserved in Chinese Medicine Museum of Beijing Yu Sheng Tang Drugstore

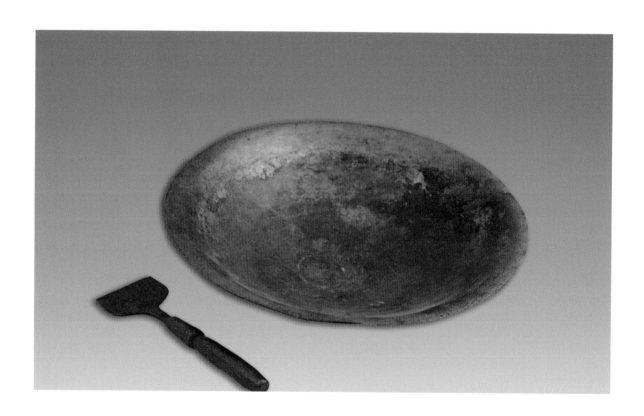

御生堂金锅铜铲

清

金质锅，铜质铲

锅：口径 36 厘米

铲柄：长 26 厘米

Gold Pot and Bronze Shovel of Yu Sheng Tang Drugstore

Qing Dynasty

Gold Pot, Bronze Shovel

Pot: Mouth Diameter 36 cm

Handle: Length 26 cm

锅：铸造，侈口，斜腹，圆底。铲：铸造，铲体厚重，铲头扁平，嵌木把手。清代御生堂用于炮制中药材的器具。

北京御生堂中医药博物馆藏

The casted pot has a widely flared mouth, an inclined belly and a round bottom. The casted shovel has a heavy body, a flat head and a wooden handle. It was used for processing and preparing medicine.

Preserved in Chinese Medicine Museum of Beijing Yu Sheng Tang Drugstore

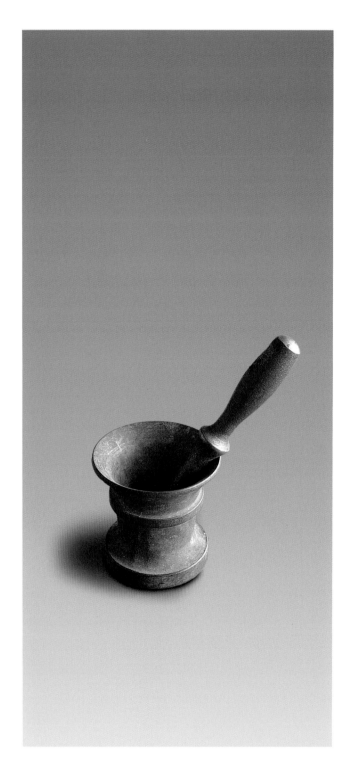

臼

清

铜质

臼：口径9.5厘米，底径8厘米，高8.5厘米

杵：长9厘米

Mortar

Qing Dynasty

Copper

Mortar: Mouth Diameter 9.5 cm/ Bottom

Diameter 8 cm/ Height 8.5 cm

Pestle: Length 9 cm

敞口，直腹，饼形足，杵中部有节与臼相印合。
由民间征集。

　成都中医药大学中医药传统文化博物馆藏

The mortar has an open mouth, an erect belly
and cake-like feet. There is a joint in the middle
part of the pestle which matches well with the
mortar. It was collected from the folk.
Preserved in Museum of Traditional Chinese
Medicine Culture, Chengdu University of Traditional
Chinese Medicine

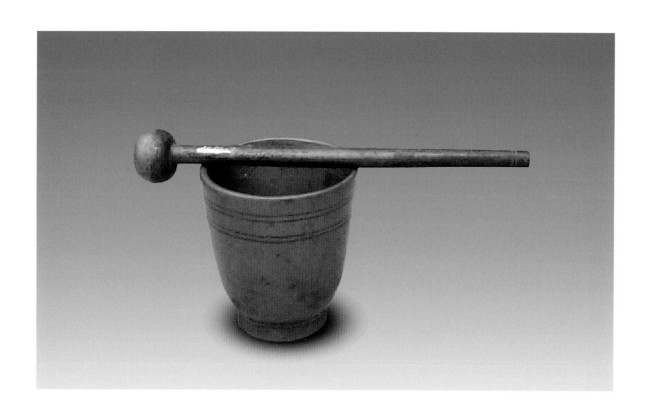

带杵药臼

清

铜质

臼：口内径 9.1 厘米，口外径 9.9 厘米，通高 10.8 厘米

杵：长 24.5 厘米，杵头径 3.3 厘米

Medicine Mortar with Pestle

Qing Dynasty

Copper

Mortar: Inner Diameter 9.1 cm/ Outer Diameter 9.9 cm/ Height 10.8 cm

Pestle: Length 24.5 cm/ Top Diameter 3.3 cm

该藏为罐形，表面光洁，饰双线纹，器物沉
稳厚重，便于使用。制药工具。1959 年入藏。
保存基本完好。

中华医学会 / 上海中医药大学医史博物馆藏

This pot-shaped mortar has a bright and clean
surface which is decorated with two-line
pattern. This heavy and stable mortar is easy
to handle. Used as a medical appliance, it was
collected in 1959 and is still in good condition.
Preserved in Chinese Medical Association/
Museum of Chinese Medicine, Shanghai
University of Traditional Chinese Medicine

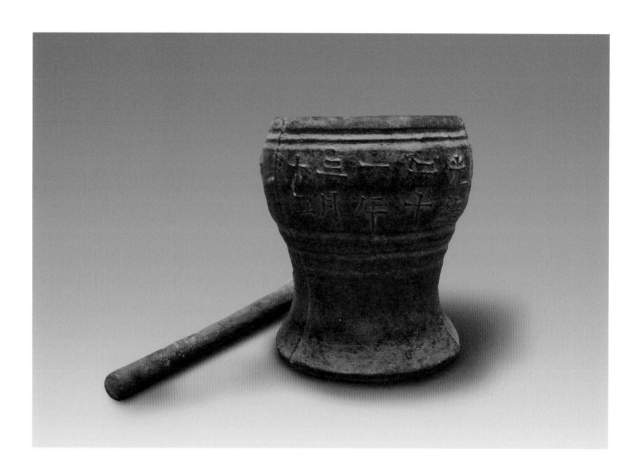

药臼

清

铁质

口径 16.3 厘米，底径 16.8 厘米，高 20.7 厘米

Medicine Mortar

Qing Dynasty

Iron

Mouth Diameter 16.3 cm/ Bottom Diameter 16.8 cm/ Height 20.7 cm

鼓腹，圈足形底，肩部及下腹部饰旋纹，腹
中部有"光绪二十一年三月十五日"铭及花
草纹饰。由民间征集。

成都中医药大学中医药传统文化博物馆藏

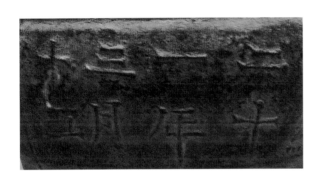

The mortar has a swelling belly and a hoop-like
leg at its bottom. The shoulder and the lower
part of the belly are decorated with vortex
pattern. Inscription "Guang Xu Er Shi Yi Nian
San Yue Shi Wu Ri" (meaning 15th March of
the 21st year of the reign of Emperor Guang
Xu) and patterns of flowers and grass are on the
middle part of the belly. It was collected from
the folk.

Preserved in Museum of Traditional Chinese
Medicine Culture, Chengdu University of Traditional
Chinese Medicine

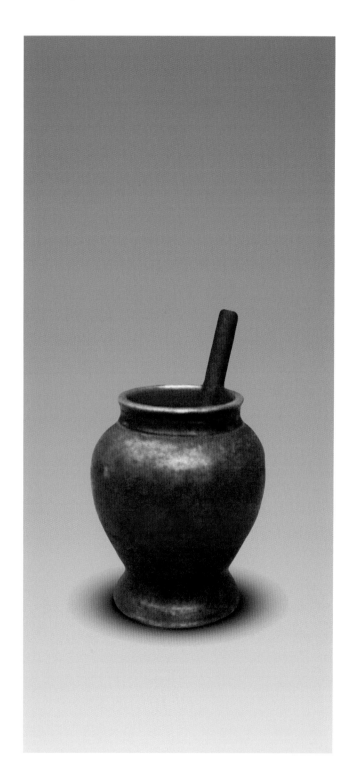

带杵药臼

清

铜质

臼：口内径 6.3 厘米，口外径 7.6 厘米，腹
径 10.5 厘米，通高 12.5 厘米

杵：长 15.8 厘米，杵头径 3.8 厘米

Medicine Mortar with Pestle

Qing Dynasty

Copper

Mortar: Inner Diameter 6.3 cm/ Outer Diameter

7.6 cm/ Belly Diameter 10.5 cm/ Height 12.5 cm

Pestle: Length 15.8 cm/ Top Diameter 3.8 cm

罐形。该藏表面光洁，腹部刻三条细纹，平底，翻沿，制作精细，器物沉稳厚重便于使用。制药工具。1959 年入藏。保存基本完好。

中华医学会 / 上海中医药大学医史博物馆藏

This pot-shaped mortar has a bright and clean surface, a belly decorated with three thin-line pattern, a flat bottom and a folded edge. This heavy and stable mortar with exquisite workmanship is easy to handle. Used as a medical appliance, it was collected in 1959 and is still in good condition.

Preserved in Chinese Medical Association/ Museum of Chinese Medicine, Shanghai University of Traditional Chinese Medicine

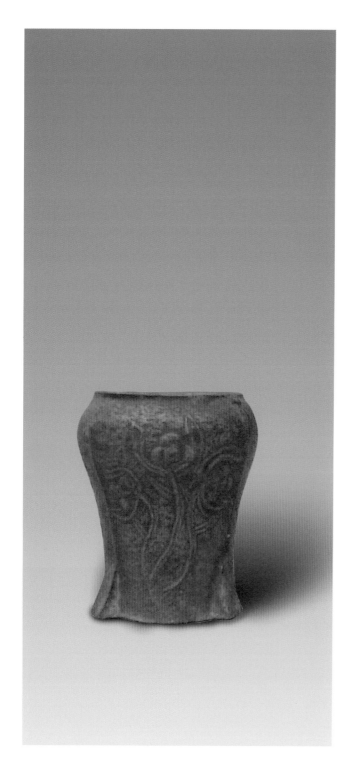

铜药臼

清

铜质

口内径 8.7 厘米，口外径 9.8 厘米，最宽径 12 厘米，底径 10.3 厘米，通高 13.8 厘米

Copper Medicine Mortar

Qing Dynasty

Copper

Inner Diameter 8.7 cm/ Outer Diameter 9.8 cm/ The Widest Diameter 12 cm/ Bottom Diameter 10.3 cm/ Height 13.8 cm

臼状。该藏平底，表面刻有花卉图案。制药
工具。1959 年入藏。保存基本完好。

中华医学会 / 上海中医药大学医史博物馆藏

This mortar has a flat bottom and flower
patterns engraved on the surface. Used as a
medical appliance, it was collected in 1959 and
is still in good condition.
Preserved in Chinese Medical Association/
Museum of Chinese Medicine, Shanghai
University of Traditional Chinese Medicine

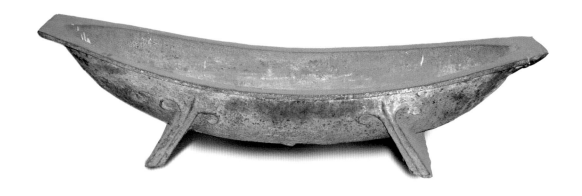

铁药碾槽

清

铁质

口长 131 厘米，口宽 31.2 厘米，通高 34 厘米

船形，两足，一头稍残，无碾饼。制药工具。陕西省咸阳市征集。

陕西医史博物馆藏

Iron Medicine Mill Groove

Qing Dynasty

Iron

Length 131 cm/ Width 31.2 cm/ Height 34 cm

The ship-like mill groove has two legs, one end slightly damaged. The mill cake is missing. It was used as a pharmaceutical appliance and was collected from Xianyang City, Shaanxi Province.

Preserved in Shaanxi Museum of Medical History

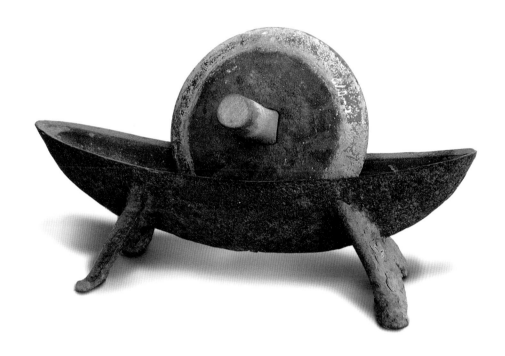

小碾槽

清

铁质

口长 44 厘米，通高 13 厘米，重 11800 克

船形，带一碾饼。完整无损。医药器具。

陕西医史博物馆藏

Small Mill Groove

Qing Dynasty

Iron

Length 44 cm/ Height 13 cm/ Weight 11,800 g

This ship-like mill grooved with a mill cake was used as a pharmaceutical appliance and is still in good shape.

Preserved in Shaanxi Museum of Medical History

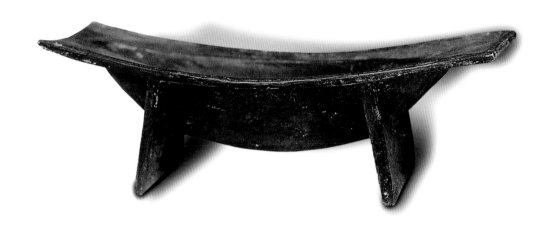

太医院药碾

清

铜质

长 26 厘米，宽 8.5 厘米，高 8 厘米

碾槽：宽 5.5 厘米，深 4 厘米

梯形扁足。制药工具。

中国国家博物馆藏

Medicine Mill of Imperial Hospital

Qing Dynasty

Copper

Length 26 cm/ Width 8.5 cm/ Height 8 cm

Mill Groove: Width 5.5 cm/ Depth 4 cm

This ladder-shaped mill with flat legs was used as a pharmaceutical appliance.

Preserved in National Museum of China

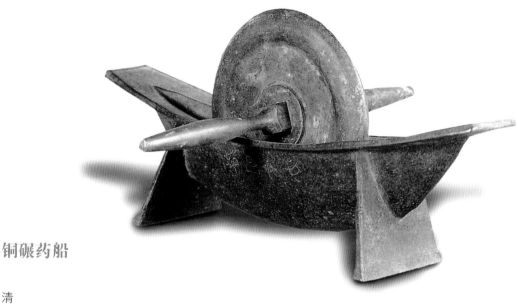

铜碾药船

清

铜质

长 32 厘米，高 8 厘米

碾槽：深 4.8 厘米

船形，暗黑色，板足。制药工具。

上海中医药博物馆藏

Ship-like Copper Medicine Mill

Qing Dynasty

Copper

Length 32 cm/ Height 8 cm

Mill Groove: Depth 4.8 cm

This dark black ship-like appliance has two board-shaped legs and was of pharmaceutical use.

Preserved in Shanghai Museum of Traditional Chinese Medicine

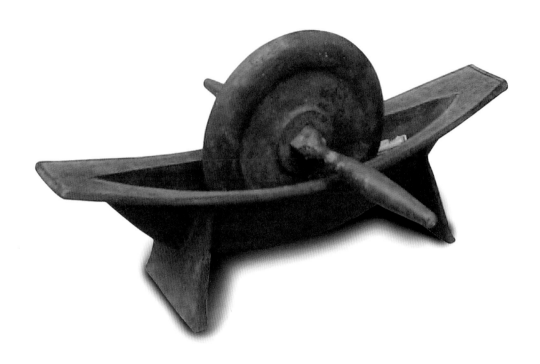

碾药船

清

铜质

通长 33 厘米，宽 8.3 厘米，高 10.1 厘米

研轮：直径 13.4 厘米，厚 1.7 厘米

Ship-like Medicine Mill

Qing Dynasty

Copper

Length 33 cm/ Width 8.3 cm/ Height 10.1 cm

Grinding Wheel：Diameter 13.4 cm/ Thickness 1.7 cm

船形。该藏用铜制成，碾轮中心有轴柄，设
计合理，坚固耐用，有使用痕迹。用于碾药。
1959 年入藏。保存基本完好。

中华医学会 / 上海中医药大学医史博物馆藏

The ship-like appliance was made of copper
with axis handles installed in the center of the
wheel, and used for grinding medicine. The
design makes the appliance strong and durable.
Traces of usage can be found on the appliance.
It was collected in 1959 and is still in good
condition.

Preserved in Chinese Medical Association/
Museum of Chinese Medicine, Shanghai
University of Traditional Chinese Medicine

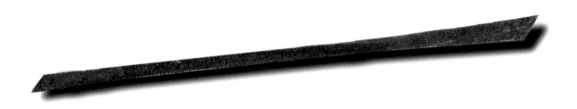

小铁刀

清

铁质

长 21 厘米，宽 0.7 厘米，重 50 克

长条形，两头为刀刃。制药工具。完整无损。

陕西医史博物馆藏

Small Iron Knife

Qing Dynasty

Iron

Length 21 cm/ Width 0.7 cm/ Weight 50 g

The long strip-like knife has two blades on both ends. It was used as a pharmaceutical appliance and is still in good shape.

Preserved in Shaanxi Museum of Medical History

小铁刀

清

铁质

长 21.5 厘米，宽 0.6 厘米，重 50 克

长条形，两头为刀刃。制药工具。完整无损。

陕西医史博物馆藏

Small Iron Knife

Qing Dynasty

Iron

Length 21.5 cm/ Width 0.6 cm/ Weight 50 g

The long strip-like knife has two blades on both ends. It was used as a pharmaceutical appliance and is still in good shape.

Preserved in Shaanxi Museum of Medical History

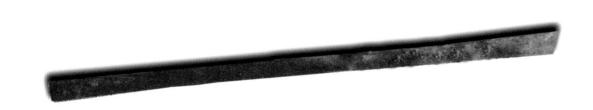

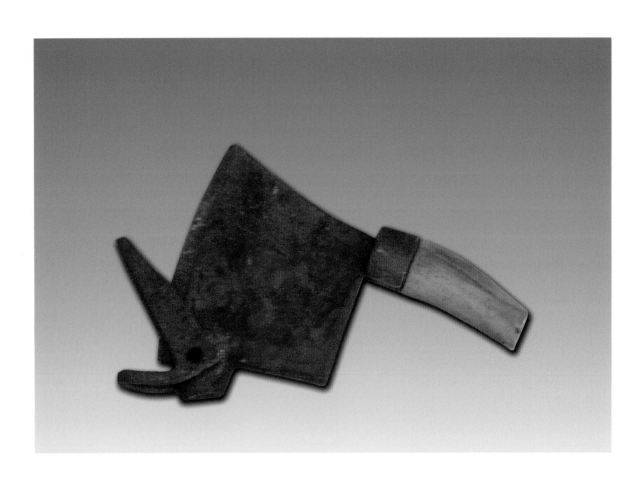

铁药刀

清

铁质

长 24 厘米，宽 17 厘米，重 700 克

Iron Medical Knife

Qing Dynasty

Iron

Length 24 cm/ Width 17 cm/ Weight 700 g

切药刀状，带一圆木把，并带一镰状铁头。苏州雷允上专用制药工具。民间征集，完整无损。

陕西医史博物馆藏

The appliance is a cutting knife with a round wooden handle and a sickle-like iron head. It was a special pharmaceutical appliance in Lei Yunshang, Suzhou. It was collected from the folk and is still in good shape.

Preserved in Shaanxi Museum of Medical History

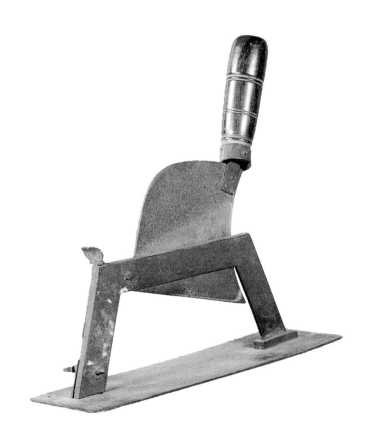

铜切药刀

清

长 19.2 厘米，通高 9.6 厘米

分刀和刀架二部分，刀把木质。制药工具。

上海中医药博物馆藏

Copper Knife for Slicing Medicine

Qing Dynasty

Length 19.2 cm/ Height 9.6 cm

This appliance is a knife with a wood-made handle and a rack for pharmaceutical use.

Preserved in Shanghai Museum of Traditional Chinese Medicine

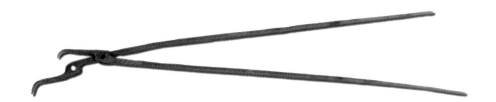

铁药钳

清

铁质

长 86 厘米，宽 3.5 厘米，重 1400 克

钳状，长柄。制药工具。完整无损。陕西省三原县征集。

陕西医史博物馆藏

Iron Medicine Tong

Qing Dynasty

Length 86 cm/ Width 3.5 cm/ Weight 1,400 g

This appliance is tong-shaped with a long handle. It was used as a pharmaceutical appliance and is still in good shape. It was collected from Sanyuan County, Shaanxi Province.

Preserved in Shaanxi Museum of Medical History

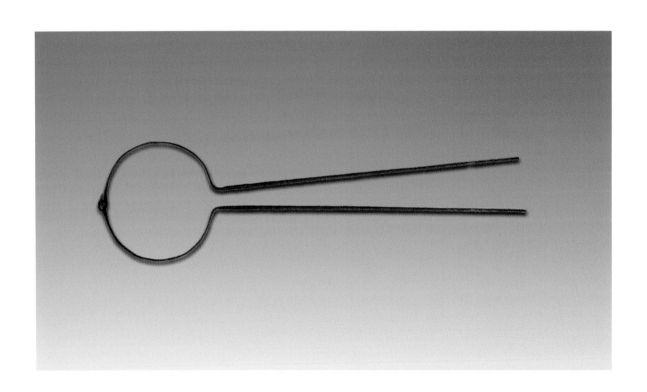

铁锻药钳

清

铁质

长 100 厘米，宽 24.5 厘米，重 1050 克

头为圆环形，把较长。制药工具。完整无损。陕西省三原县征集。

陕西医史博物馆藏

Iron-forged Medicine Tong

Qing Dynasty

Iron

Length 100 cm/ Width 24.5 cm/ Weight 1,050 g

The tong has a ring-like head and a long handle. It was used as a pharmaceutical appliance and is still in good shape. It was collected from Sanyuan County, Shaanxi Province.

Preserved in Shaanxi Museum of Medical History

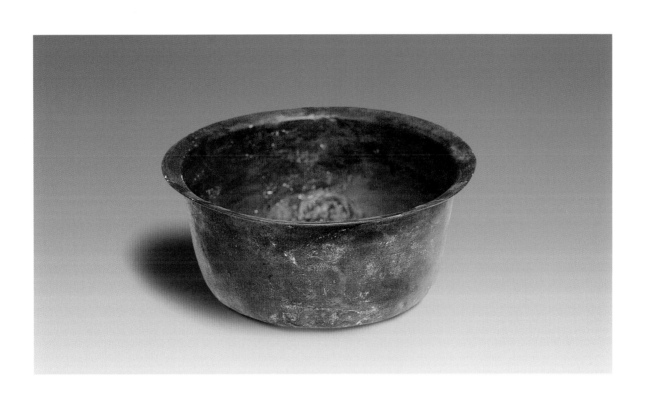

太医院药锅

清

铜质

口径 26 厘米，底径 22 厘米，高 14 厘米

侈口，直腹，平底。煎洗药物用具。

故宫博物院藏

Medicine Cauldron of Imperial Hospital

Qing Dynasty

Copper

Mouth Diameter 26 cm/ Bottom Diameter 22 cm/ Height 14 cm

This is a medicine cauldron with a wide flared mouth, a straight belly and a flat bottom. It is used for decocting Chinese medicine and washing and disinfecting medical implements.

Preserved in The Palace Museum

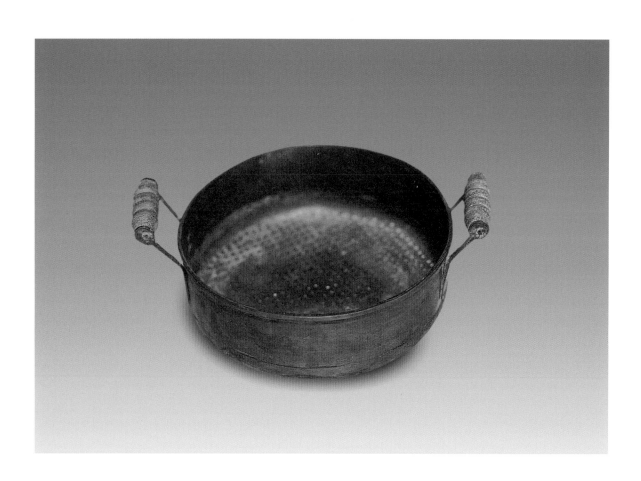

太医院双耳药筛

清

铜质

直径 15.5 厘米，高 8 厘米

Two-Handle Medicine Sieve of Imperial Hospital

Qing Dynasty

Copper

Diameter 15.5 cm/ Height 8 cm

生产加工药物工具，根据筛孔的大小筛选药

末的粒度。

故宫博物院藏

This sieve is used for producing and processing medicines. Particles are screened by different sieve meshes.

Preserved in The Palace Museum

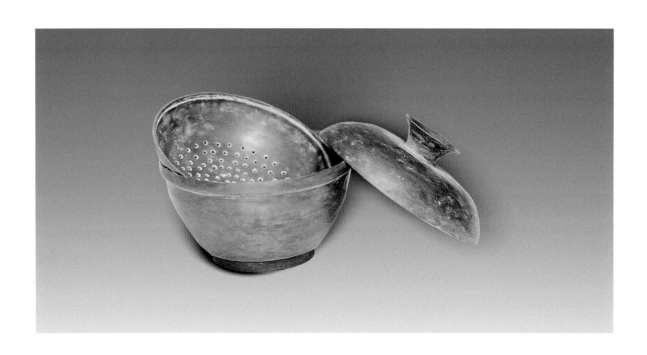

太医院盖碗药筛

清

锡质

底碗：直径 12.5 厘米，高 6.5 厘米

筛：直径 12 厘米，高 3.5 厘米

盖：直径 12 厘米，高 4 厘米

Medicine Sieve Bowl with Cover of Imperial Hospital

Qing Dynasty

Tin

Bowl: Diameter 12.5 cm/ Height 6.5 cm

Sieve: Diameter 12 cm/ Height 3.5 cm

Cover: Diameter 12 cm/ Height 4 cm

一套三件，子母口。用于生产加工药物，筛
选药末的粒度。

故宫博物院藏

This three-piece medical implement consists of
a sieve, a bowl and a snap cover. It was used
to produce and process medications and screen
them into various sizes.
Preserved in The Palace Museum

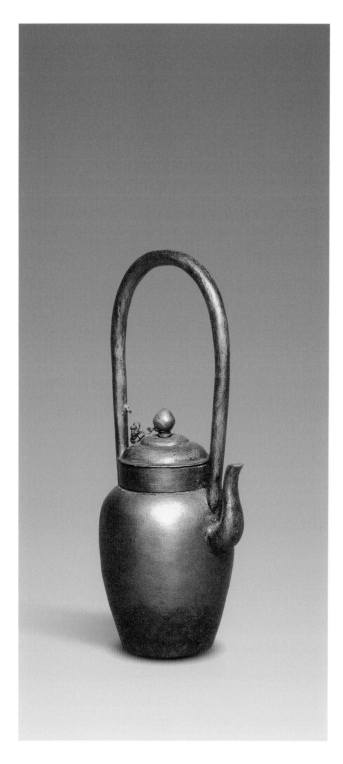

御药房温药壶

清

银质

口径 5.5 厘米，腹径 9 厘米，高 26 厘米

Medicine Heating Pot of Imperial Pharmacy

Qing Dynasty

Silver

Mouth Diameter 5.5 cm/ Belly Diameter 9 cm/

Height 26 cm

壶腹外壁刻有"御药房"字样。

故宫博物院藏

Characters "Yu Yao Fang", which mean the
imperial pharmacy, were carved on the outer
wall of the pot belly.

Preserved in The Palace Museum

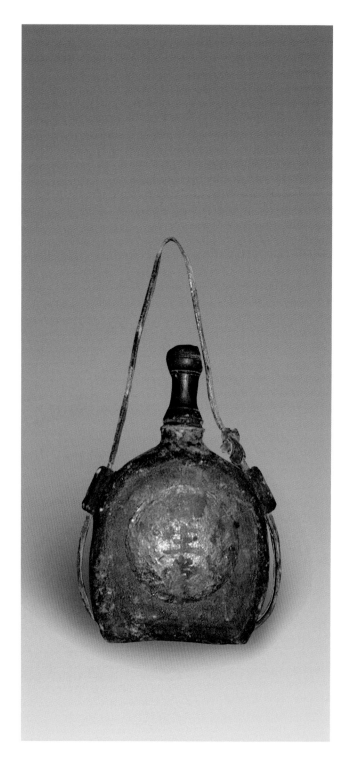

御生堂药酒壶

清

锡质

腹径 23 厘米，通高 38 厘米

底：长 15 厘米，宽 8 厘米

提手：26 厘米

Medical Wine Pot of Yu Sheng Tang

Qing Dynasty

Tin

Belly Diameter 23 cm/ Height 38 cm

Bottom: Length 15 cm/ Width 8 cm

Handle: Length 26 cm

直口，短颈，溜肩，肩上附耳，耳中有提手穿过，平底，带盖。正、反两面都有"御生堂"的字号，壶内为锡质，外包一层兽皮。1992年，内蒙古牧民家征集。

北京御生堂中医药博物馆藏

The pot has a straight mouth, a short neck, a flat bottom, a lid, a sloping shoulder with ears and two lifting handles through them. The inscriptions of "Yu Sheng Tang" can be seen on both sides. The interior is made of tin while the exterior is covered with animal skin. This pot was collected from an Inner Mongolian herdsman's family in 1992.

Preserved in Chinese Medicine Museum of Beijing Yu Sheng Tang Drugstore

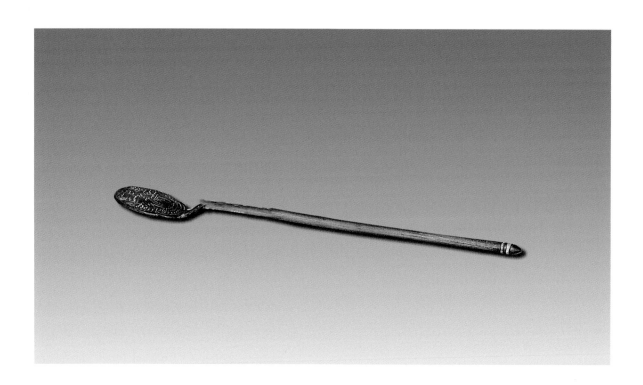

铜药匙

清

铜质

长 18.5 厘米，宽 2.5 厘米，重 50 克

Copper Medicine Spoon

Qing Dynasty

Copper

Length 18.5 cm/ Width 2.5 cm/ Weight 50 g

匙头呈圆形，柄为长圆形。药具。完整无损。

陕西医史博物馆藏

The medicine spoon has a round head and a cylindrical handle. This spoon was used as a medicine tool and is preserved in good condition.

Preserved in Shaanxi Museum of Medical History

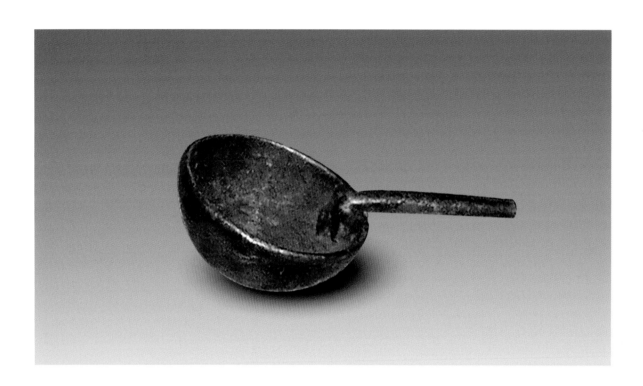

铜药勺头

清

铜质

口径 2 厘米，长 3.5 厘米，重 1 克

Head of Copper Medicine Spoon

Qing Dynasty

Copper

Mouth Diameter 2 cm/ Length 3.5 cm/ Weight 1 g

勺小巧，勺头深，勺柄细短。药具。完整无损。

内蒙古自治区中蒙医研究所征集。

陕西医史博物馆藏

This tiny spoon has a deep head and a thin and short handle. It was used as a medicine tool and is preserved in good condition. The spoon was collected by Institute for Chinese and Mongolian Medical Science, the Inner Mongolia Autonomous Region.

Preserved in Shaanxi Museum of Medical History

勺

清

铜质

长 11 厘米

由民间征集。

成都中医药大学中医药传统文化博物馆藏

Spoon

Qing Dynasty

Copper

Length 11 cm

This spoon was collected from the folk.

Preserved in Museum of Traditional Chinese Medicine Culture, Chengdu University of Traditional Chinese Medicine

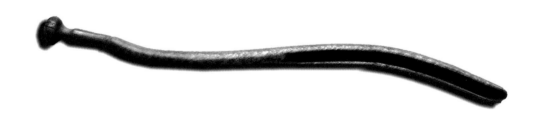

匙

清

铜质

长 16 厘米

尾部圆钝，头部为圆圈形。由民间征集。

成都中医药大学中医药传统文化博物馆藏

Spoon

Qing Dynasty

Copper

Length 16 cm

The spoon has a circular head and a blunt closed end. It was collected from the folk.

Preserved in Museum of Traditional Chinese Medicine Culture, Chengdu University of Traditional Chinese Medicine

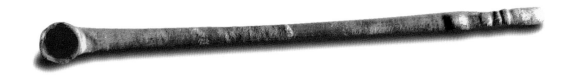

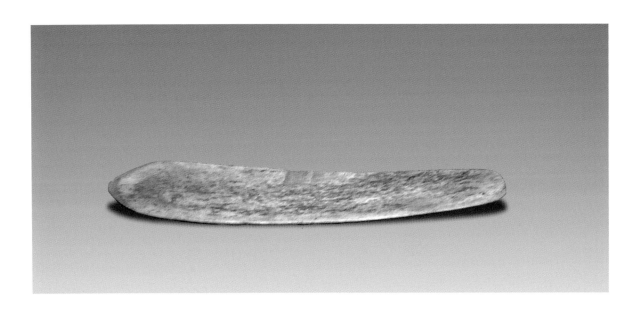

匕

清

铜质

长 8.5 厘米

由民间征集。

成都中医药大学中医药传统文化博物馆藏

An Ancient Type of Spoon

Qing Dynasty

Copper

Length 8.5 cm

The spoon was collected from the folk.

Preserved in Museum of Traditional Chinese Medicine Culture, Chengdu University of Traditional Chinese Medicine

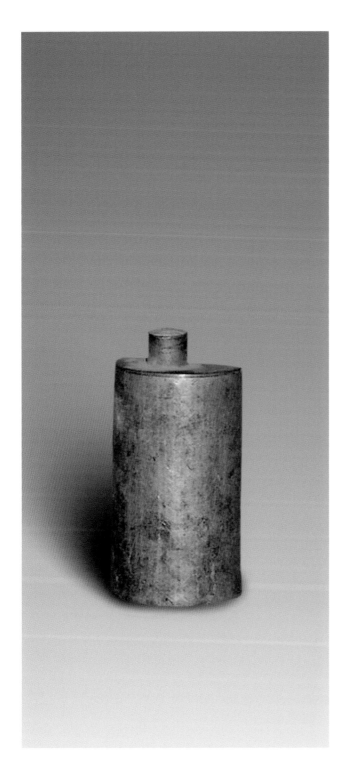

铜半圆药瓶

清

铜质

口径 0.6 厘米，底径 3 厘米，通高 5.5 厘米，

重 50 克

直口，腹为半圆，平底。贮药器具。完整无损。

陕西医史博物馆藏

Copper Semicircular Medicine Bottle

Qing Dynasty

Copper

Mouth Diameter 0.6 cm/ Bottom Diameter 3 cm/

Height 5.5 cm/ Weight 50 g

The medicine bottle has a straight mouth, a semicircular belly and a flat bottom. It was used for storing medicine and is preserved in good condition.

Preserved in Shaanxi Museum of Medical History

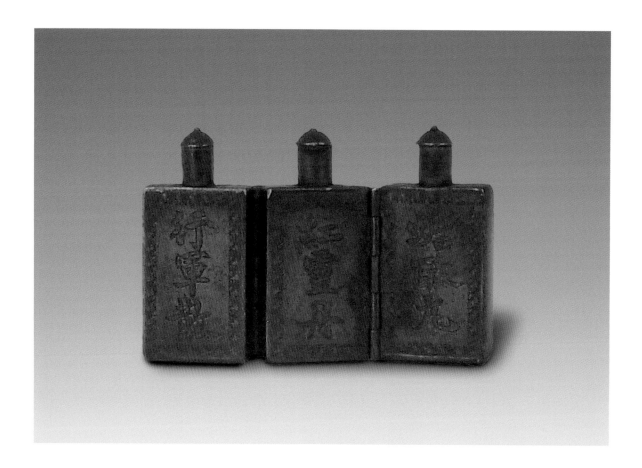

链环药瓶

清

铜质

总长 5.1 厘米，单瓶宽 1.7 厘米，厚 0.6 厘米，高 3.5 厘米

Medicine Bottles Connected with Hinges

Qing Dynasty

Copper

Total Length 5.1 cm/ Width of Each Bottle 1.7 cm/ Thickness 0.6 cm/ Height 3.5 cm

扁方形。该藏为三个相同大小的单体瓶连结
而成。瓶身一面分别浅刻有"行军散""红
灵丹""蟾酥丸"字样，另面浅刻草药图案，
雕刻精细，表面光亮。便于携带。盛药用。
1954 年入藏。保存基本完好。

中华医学会 / 上海中医药大学医史博物馆藏

This flattened square medicine container
consists of three bottles of the same size. On
one side of the medicine bottle, it is shallowly
engraved with the names of traditional Chinese
medicine "Xing Jun San" "Hong Ling Dan"
and "Chan Su Wan", while the other side is
decorated shallowly with the pattern of herbs.
The surface of the bottle is bright and smooth,
and it is carved exquisitely. This medicine bottle
set is easy to carry, and was used for storing
medicine. It was collected in the year 1954 and
is preserved in basically good condition.
Preserved in Chinese Medical Association/
Museum of Chinese Medicine, Shanghai
University of Traditional Chinese Medicine

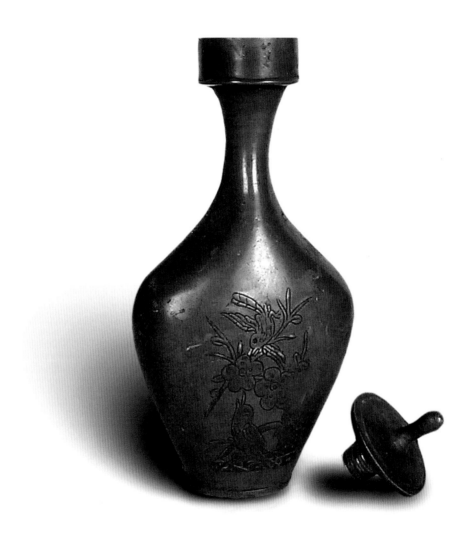

长颈扁药瓶

清

铜质

口内径 1.5 厘米，口外径 3.6 厘米，宽 8.5 厘米，厚 4.6 厘米，通高 18.5 厘米

扁瓶形。该藏表面光滑，一面雕有花鸟图案，上有螺旋口带钮瓶盖，封闭严密。瓶底款识待考。医用。1954 年入藏。保存基本完好。

中华医学会 / 上海中医药大学医史博物馆藏

Flattened Medicine Bottle with a Long Neck

Qing Dynasty

Copper

Inner Diameter 1.5 cm/ Outer Diameter 3.6 cm/ Width 8.5 cm/ Thickness 4.6 cm/ Height 18.5 cm

This flattened medicine bottle has a smooth surface and a helical mouth with knob cover which keeps the bottle air tight. One side of the bottle is engraved with the patterns of flowers and birds. The inscription on the bottom remains to be investigated. This bottle was for medical use and was collected in the year 1954. It is preserved in basically good condition.

Preserved in Chinese Medical Association/Museum of Chinese Medicine, Shanghai University of Traditional Chinese Medicine

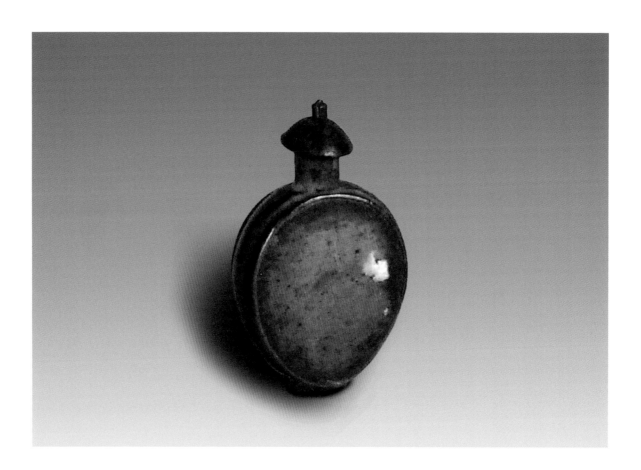

铜药瓶

清

铜质

口外径 0.52 厘米，宽 2.15 厘米，厚 0.85 厘米，通高 3.45 厘米

Coppery Medicine Bottle

Qing Dynasty

Copper

Outer Diameter 0.52 cm/ Width 2.15 cm/ Thickness 0.85 cm/ Height 3.45 cm

扁瓶状。该藏表面光滑，工艺精细，上有螺旋口带钮瓶盖，专门用于存放散剂。医用药瓶。1954 年入藏。保存基本完好。

中华医学会 / 上海中医药大学医史博物馆藏

The flattened medicine bottle has a smooth surface and a helical mouth with knob cover. It is made in exquisite workmanship, and was particularly used for storing pulvis. The medicine bottle was collected in 1954 and is preserved in basically good condition.

Preserved in Chinese Medical Association/ Museum of Chinese Medicine, Shanghai University of Traditional Chinese Medicine

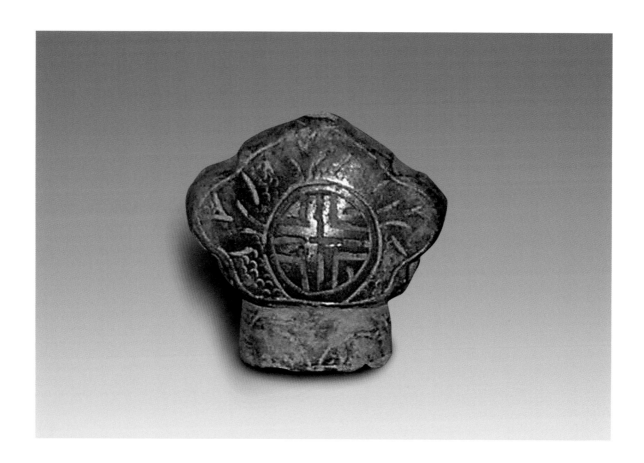

铜扁药瓶

清

铜质

口径 0.25 厘米，底径 0.4 厘米，通高 3.6 厘米，重 50 克

Copper Flattened Medicine Bottle

Qing Dynasty

Copper

Mouth Diameter 0.25 cm/ Bottom Diameter 0.4 cm/ Height 3.6 cm/ Weight 50 g

半圆，腹为椭圆状，有纹饰。贮药器具。有残。

陕西医史博物馆藏

The semicircular medicine bottle has an oval belly decorated with patterns. It was used for storing medicine and is slightly damaged.

Preserved in Shaanxi Museum of Medical History

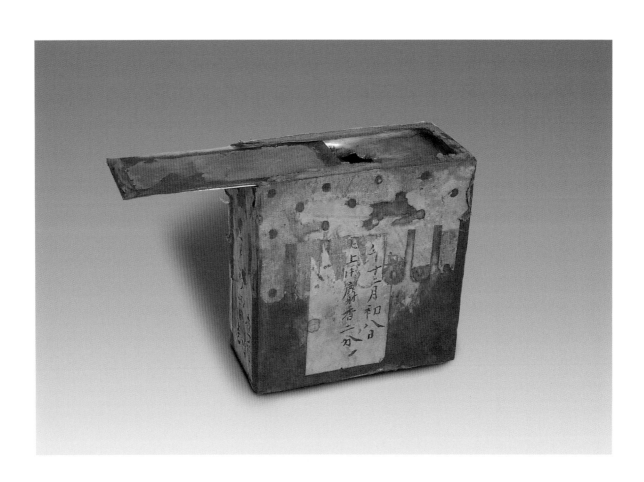

麝香银盒

清

银质

宽 8.9 厘米，厚 4 厘米，高 8.7 厘米

Silver Box for Musk

Qing Dynasty

Silver

Width 8.9 cm/ Thickness 4 cm/ Height 8.7 cm

方形，用于盛放麝香。该藏有抽拉式盒盖，盖外侧有包布以防麝香味溢出，现包布撕开，盒盖下面被凿开，洞口不规则。盒空。盒身贴两纸标签，上书"□月初四封　查看""□年十二月初八日□上用麝香二分"等字样，盒底有款。1986 年入藏，原藏故宫博物院。外部保存基本完好。

中华医学会 / 上海中医药大学医史博物馆藏

The square silver box was used for holding musk. It has a pull-out cover, wrapped with cloth outside in case that the fragrance of musk overflows. Now, the cloth is torn apart, while the underside of the cover is chiseled with an irregular hole. The box is empty. There are two paper labels stuck on the body of the box, recording the dates of use. On the bottom of the silver box, an inscription is carved. The box was collected in 1986 and was originally Preserved in The Palace Museum. The outer part of the box is kept in basically good condition, and its underside of the cover is chiseled .

Preserved in Chinese Medical Association/ Museum of Chinese Medicine, Shanghai University of Traditional Chinese Medicine

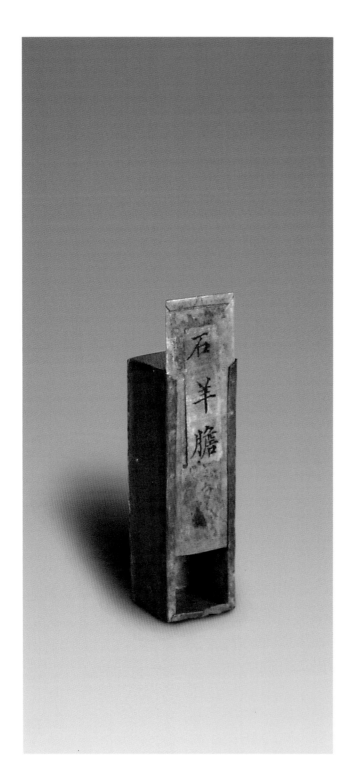

药盒

清

银质

宽 1.8 厘米，厚 1.5 厘米，通高 5.1 厘米

Medicine Box

Qing Dynasty

Silver

Width 1.8 cm/ Thickness 1.5 cm/ Height 5.1 cm

方形，用于盛药。为馆内收藏的一组石羊胆
药盒之一，银皮制作，工艺粗糙，抽拉式板
状盒盖，盖上粘有"石羊胆"黄色标记。
1986 年入藏。保存基本完好。

中华医学会 / 上海中医药大学医史博物馆藏

The square medicine box was used for holding
medicine. It is one of a set of "Shi Yang Dan"
medicine boxes collected by the museum.
This silver-skinned box is made in rough
workmanship and has a pull-out plate-like
cover, stuck with a yellow tag marking "Shi
Yang Dan". It was collected in 1986.
Preserved in Chinese Medical Association/
Museum of Chinese Medicine, Shanghai
University of Traditional Chinese Medicine

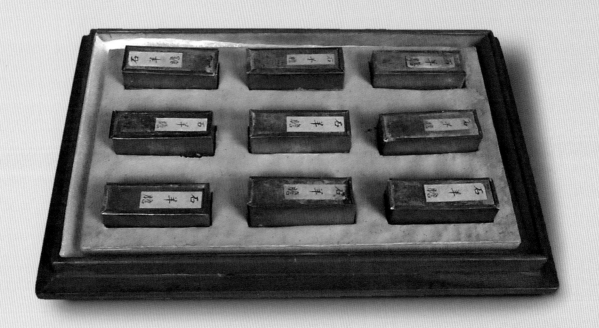

药盒

清

银质

Medicine Box

Qing Dynasty

Silver

方形，用于盛药。一组（共 9 只）石羊胆药
盒用木盒套装，小药盒用银皮制作，工艺粗
糙，抽拉式板状盒盖，盖上粘有"石羊胆"
黄色标记。1986 年入藏。

中华医学会 / 上海中医药大学医史博物馆藏

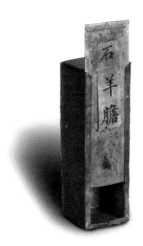

The square medicine box was used for holding
medicine. It is a set of "Shi Yang Dan" medicine
boxes (with a total number of 9 boxes) held by
a wooden box. These silver-skinned boxes are
made in rough workmanship and have pull-
out plate-like covers, stuck with a yellow tag
marking "Shi Yang Dan". It was collected in
1986.

Preserved in Chinese Medical Association/
Museum of Chinese Medicine, Shanghai
University of Traditional Chinese Medicine

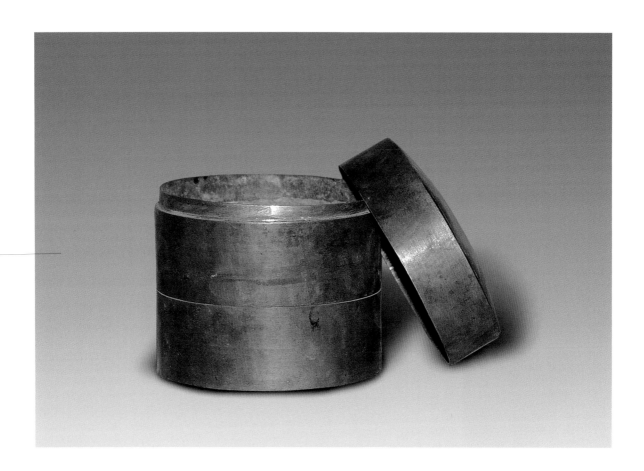

铜药盒

清

铜质

口径 7.8 厘米，底径 7.8 厘米，通高 7.7 厘米，重 350 克

Copper Medicine Box

Qing Dynasty

Copper

Mouth Diameter 7.8 cm/ Bottom Diameter 7.8 cm/ Height 7.7 cm/ Weight 350 g

子母口，直腹，圈足，盒分三部分：盖、中层、底层。贮药器具。完整无损。陕西省咸阳市征集。

陕西医史博物馆藏

The medicine box has a snap-lid, a straight belly and a ring foot. It is composed of three parts: the cover, the middle layer and the bottom layer. It was used for storing medicine and is preserved in good condition. The medicine box was collected from Xianyang City, Shaanxi Province.

Preserved in Shaanxi Museum of Medical History

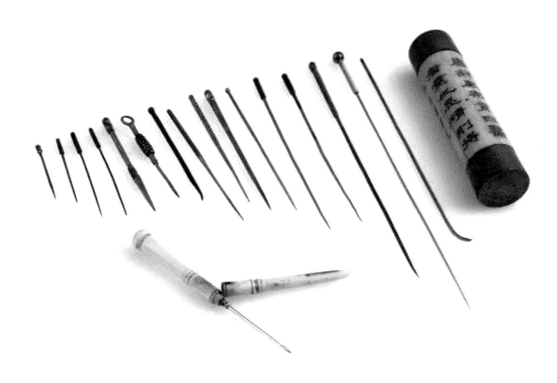

御生堂针具

清

金属

长 4~16 厘米

Acupuncture Needles from Yu Sheng Tang Drugstore

Qing Dynasty

Metal

Length 4–16 cm

御生堂御医在宫中所用针灸用具。形态多样，有金针、银针等各种贵金属针具。附圆柱形针筒，筒身刻"唐许胤宗书曰医者意也思精则得之……"。

北京御生堂中医药博物馆藏

These needles were used by the imperial physicians in the imperial palace. There are various kinds of needles, including the gold and silver ones. The body of cylindrical container was carved with the inscriptions meaning "only the skillful physicians deserve to have it, written by Xu Yinzong of the Tang Dynasty".
Preserved in Chinese Medicine Museum of Beijing Yu Sheng Tang Drugstore

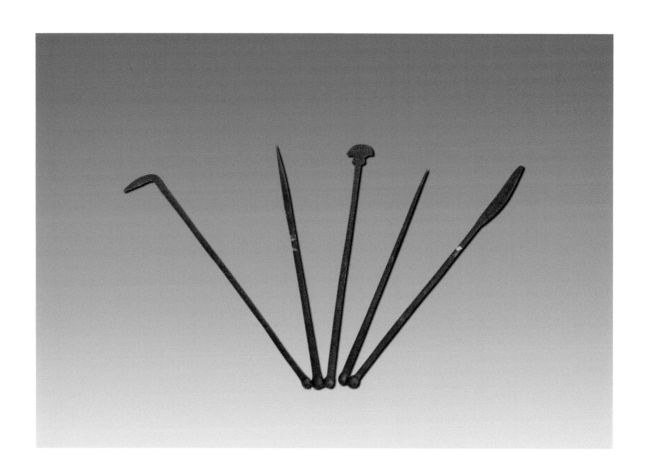

外科手术器械

清

铁质

长 12.5 厘米，重 50 克

Surgical Instruments

Qing Dynasty

Iron

Length 12.5 cm/ Weight 50 g

三棱针、圆勾针状、镰形器、长勺、小铲等。

医疗器械。完整无损。陕西省澄城县征集。

陕西医史博物馆藏

These are a series of surgical instruments, including a three-edged needle, a circular hook-like needle, a sickle-like instrument, a long spoon, and a small scoop. They are preserved in good condition and were collected from Chengcheng County, Shaanxi Province.

Preserved in Shaanxi Museum of Medical History

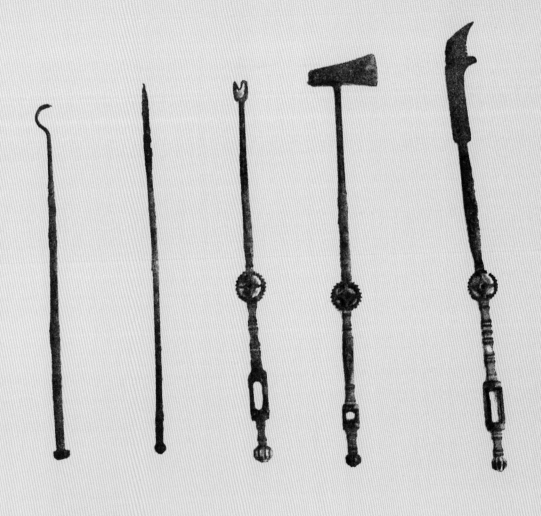

中医外科器械

清

黄铜质

刀：长 13.2 厘米

斧：长 12.5 厘米

双钩：长 11.5 厘米

矛：长 11 厘米

单钩：长 10.9 厘米

陕西泾阳李明廉医生祖传遗物，共五件，系仿照我国传统兵器制成。斧、双钩、刀柄有镂空花饰。

陕西医史博物馆藏

Traditional Chinese Surgical Instruments

Qing Dynasty

Copper

Knife: Length 13.2 cm

Axe: Length 12.5 cm

Double Hook: Length 11.5 cm

Spear: Length 11 cm

Single Hook: Length 10.9 cm

These traditional Chinese surgical instruments are ancestral remains of Doctor Li Minglian in Jingyang County, Shaanxi Province. There are five instruments imitating traditional Chinese weapons. Hollow patterns are decorated on the handles of the axe, the double hook and the hilt.

Preserved in Shaanxi Museum of Medical History

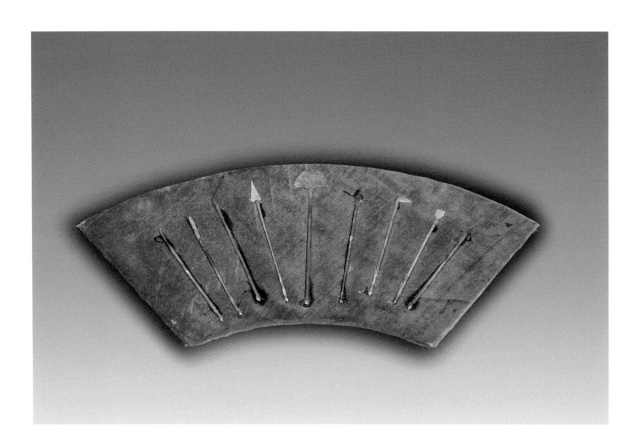

外科器具

清

铁质

九件分别长：11.5 厘米，10 厘米，10 厘米，12.2 厘米，13.5 厘米，11.4 厘米，10.1 厘米，10.6 厘米，9.2 厘米

Surgical Instruments

Qing Dynasty

Iron

Length of the 9 Instruments: 11.5 cm, 10 cm, 10 cm, 12.2 cm, 13.5 cm, 11.4 cm, 10.1 cm, 10.6 cm, 9.2 cm

一套九件：钩针、药匙、三棱针、大烙铁、大铲、小烙铁、镰刀、小铲、三棱针。医用外科器具。完整无损。陕西省西安市临潼区征集。

陕西医史博物馆藏

This set is composed of 9 instruments, including small scoop, medicine spoon, hook, big soldering iron, small soldering iron, sickle and three-edged needle. They were used as medical surgical instruments and are preserved in good condition. They were collected from Lintong District, Xi'an City, Shaanxi Province.

Preserved in Shaanxi Museum of Medical History

中医外科用具

清末

铜质

最长 25 厘米，最短 11.5 厘米

包括刀、剪、镊、探针、药勺等 35 种。系北京鲁氏老中医家传四代之物。

北京中医药大学中医药博物馆藏

Traditional Chinese Surgical Instruments

Late Qing Dynasty

Copper

The Longest: Length 25 cm/ The Shortest: Length 11.5 cm

This set is composed of 35 instruments, including scalpel, scissors, tweezers, probe, and medicine spoon. It is a 4-generation heirloom of the Lu's, a family of traditional Chinese medicine in Beijing.

Preserved in Museum of Chinese Medicine, Beijing University of Chinese Medicine

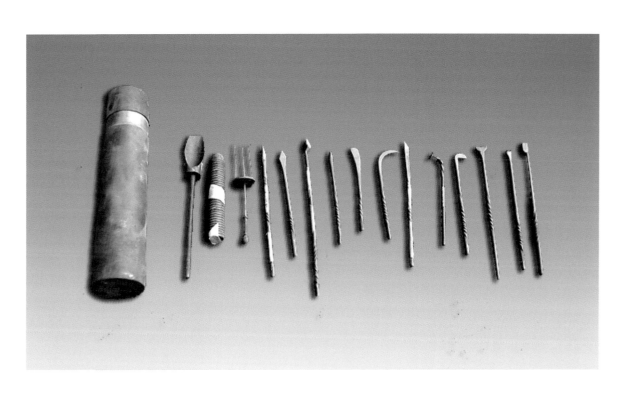

手术器具

Surgical Instruments

清

铜质

手术器具一套，15 件组合。

江苏省中医药博物馆藏

Qing Dynasty

Copper

This set is composed of 15 instruments.

Preserved in Jiangsu Museum of Traditional

Chinese Medicine

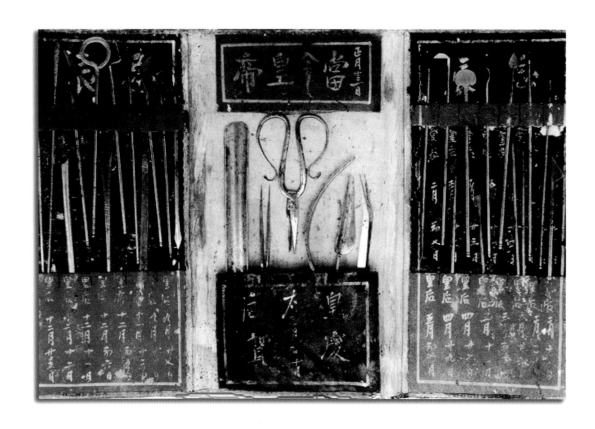

中医外科器械

清

33 件套，置于专用皮革外套中。套内书有"皇太后庆贺"并记有帝后等的"忌辰"。

伦敦科学博物馆藏

Traditional Chinese Surgical Instruments

Qing Dynasty

This set is composed of 33 instruments. It is put in appropriative leather sheath, with the records of "Huang Tai Hou Qing He" (congratulations from the Empress Dowager) and the death days of the kings, the queens, etc. on the inside.

Preserved in Science Museum, London

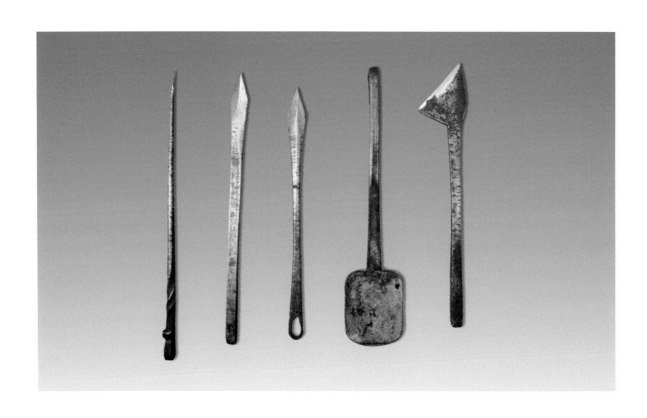

铁质小针、刀、铜匙

清

铁质

针、刀：分别长 10~12 厘米

铜匙：长 10.5 厘米

Iron Needles, Knife and Copper Spoon

Qing Dynasty

Iron

Needles and Knife: Length 10–12 cm

Spoon: Length 10.5 cm

清代中晚期医用器具，为此期中医发展较为
成熟的医用工具，主要用于外科。一套五件，
分别为三针、一刀、一铲形铜匙。

张雅宗藏

These five pieces, medical appliances of the
Late Qing Dynasty, consist of three needles,
one knife and one spade-shaped spoon. As the
surgical instruments, they represent the mature
development of Chinese Medical appliance in
the Mid-Late Qing Dynasty.
Collected by Zhang Yazong

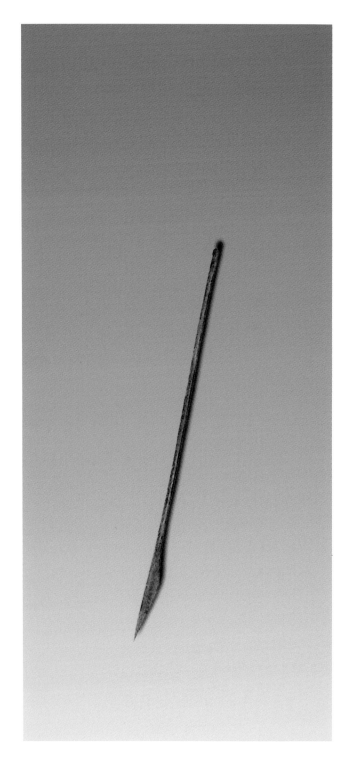

外科斜刃刀

清

铁质

通长 12.3 厘米

柄：径 0.3 厘米

刃：长 1.9 厘米

Surgical Scalpel with Oblique Blade

Qing Dynasty

Iron

Length 12.3 cm

Hilt: Diameter 0.3 cm

Blade: Length 1.9 cm

直形，为外科手术用具。斜刃刀是中医外科
最基本的手术用具，主要用做切开疮痈。这
是该馆通过自购、征集、受捐等方式收藏展
出的 78 件清末中医外科手术用具之一。保
存基本完好，钩尖处有使用痕迹，手柄处有
轻微锈斑。

中华医学会 / 上海中医药大学医史博物馆藏

The straight scalpel was used as a surgical
instrument. Surgical scalpels with oblique blade
are the most basic surgical instrument used to
incise skin ulcer. This is one of the 78 exhibited
traditional Chinese medical surgical instruments
in the late Qing Dynasty. They were collected
through purchasing, solicitation, donation, etc.
It is preserved in basically good condition.
The point of the hook shows sign of use, while
slight rust appears on the hilt.
Preserved in Chinese Medical Association/
Museum of Chinese Medicine, Shanghai
University of Traditional Chinese Medicine

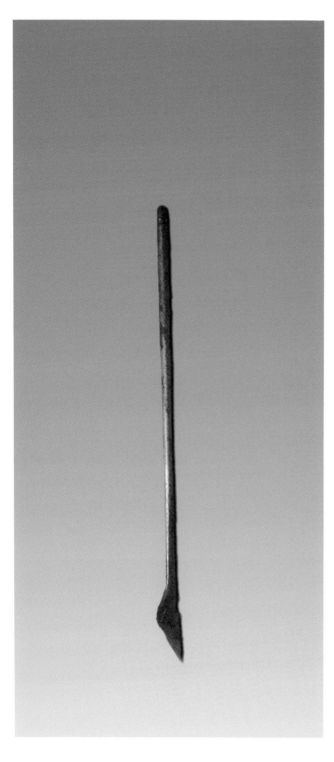

外科斜刃刀

清

铁质

通长 13.65 厘米

柄：径 0.3 厘米

刃：长 1.8 厘米

Surgical Scalpel with Oblique Blade

Qing Dynasty

Iron

Length 13.65 cm

Hilt: Diameter 0.3 cm

Blade: Length 1.8 cm

直形，为外科手术用具。斜刃刀是中医外科
最基本的手术用具，主要用做切开疮痈。这
是该馆通过接受卢大均中医师捐献而收藏的
一组清末中医外科手术用具之一。保存基本
完好，钩尖处有使用痕迹，手柄处有轻微锈斑。

中华医学会／上海中医药大学医史博物馆藏

The straight scalpel was used as a surgical
instrument. Surgical scalpels with oblique
blade are the most basic surgical instrument for
incising skin ulcer. This is one of a series of
traditional Chinese medical surgical instruments
in the late Qing Dynasty donated by practitioner
Lu Dajun of traditional Chinese medicine. It is
preserved in basically good condition. The point
of the hook shows sign of use, while slight rust
appears on the hilt.

Preserved in Chinese Medical Association/
Museum of Chinese Medicine, Shanghai
University of Traditional Chinese Medicine

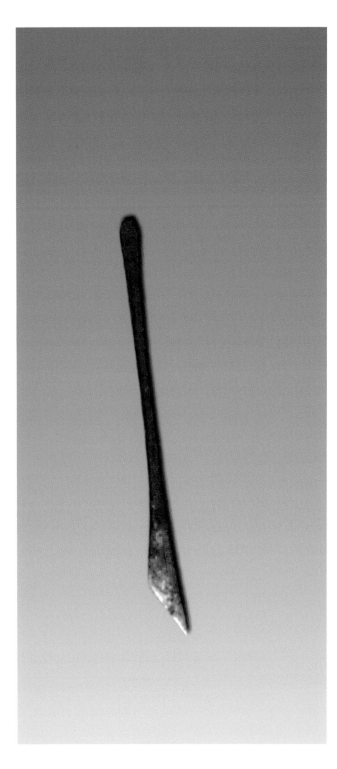

外科斜刃刀

清

铁质

通长 6.3 厘米

柄：宽 0.2 厘米

刃：长 1.1 厘米

Surgical Scalpel with Oblique Blade

Qing Dynasty

Iron

Length 6.3 cm

Hilt: Width 0.2 cm

Blade: Length 1.1 cm

直形，为外科手术用具。斜刃刀是中医外科
最基本的手术用具，主要用做切开疮痈。这
是该馆通过自购、征集、受捐等方式收藏展
出的 78 件清末中医外科手术用具之一。保
存基本完好，钩尖处有使用痕迹，手柄处有
轻微锈斑。

中华医学会 / 上海中医药大学医史博物馆藏

The straight scalpel was used as a surgical
instrument. Surgical scalpels with oblique
blade are the most basic surgical instrument
for incising skin ulcer. This is one of the 78
exhibited traditional Chinese medical surgical
instruments in the late Qing Dynasty collected
by purchasing, solicitation, donation, etc. It is
preserved in basically good condition. The point
of the hook shows sign of use, while slight rust
appears on the hilt.

Preserved in Chinese Medical Association/
Museum of Chinese Medicine, Shanghai
University of Traditional Chinese Medicine

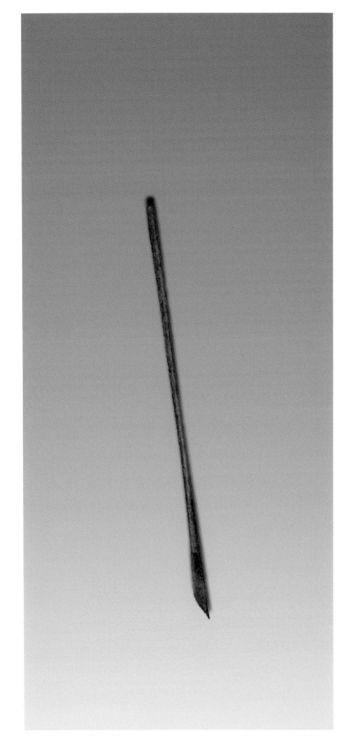

外科斜刃刀

清

铁质

通长 8.7 厘米

柄：宽 0.2 厘米

刃：长 0.7 厘米

Surgical Scalpel with Oblique Blade

Qing Dynasty

Iron

Length 8.7 cm

Hilt: Width 0.2 cm

Blade: Length 0.7 cm

直形，为外科手术用具。斜刃刀是中医外科
最基本的手术用具，主要用做切开疮痈。这
是该馆通过自购、征集、受捐等方式收藏展
出的 78 件清末中医外科手术用具之一。保
存基本完好，钩尖处有使用痕迹，手柄处有
轻微锈斑。

中华医学会 / 上海中医药大学医史博物馆藏

The straight scalpel was used as a surgical
instrument. Surgical scalpels with oblique
blade are the most basic surgical instrument
for incising skin ulcer. This is one of the 78
exhibited traditional Chinese medical surgical
instruments in the late Qing Dynasty collected
through purchasing, solicitation, donation, etc.
It is preserved in basically good condition.
The point of the hook shows sign of use, while
slight rust appears on the hilt.
Preserved in Chinese Medical Association/
Museum of Chinese Medicine, Shanghai
University of Traditional Chinese Medicine

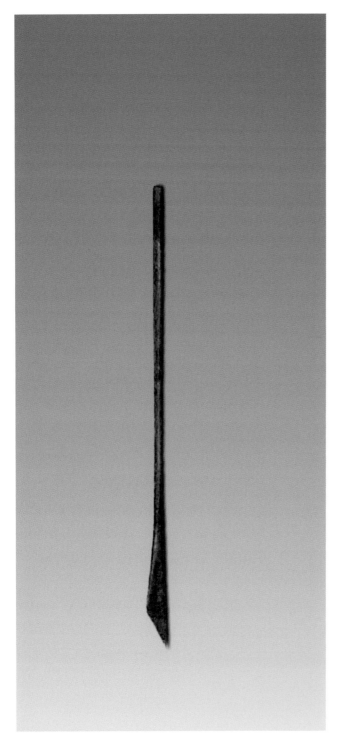

外科斜刃刀

清

铁质

通长 8.5 厘米

柄：宽 0.2 厘米

刃：长 0.7 厘米

Surgical Scalpel with Oblique Blade

Qing Dynasty

Iron

Length 8.5 cm

Hilt: Width 0.2 cm

Blade: Length 0.7 cm

直形，为外科手术用具。斜刃刀是中医外科最基本的手术用具，主要用做切开疮痈。这是该馆通过自购、征集、受捐等方式收藏展出的 78 件清末中医外科手术用具之一。保存基本完好，钩尖处有使用痕迹，手柄处有轻微锈斑。

中华医学会 / 上海中医药大学医史博物馆藏

The straight scalpel was used as a surgical instrument. Surgical scalpels with oblique blade are the most basic surgical instrument for incising skin ulcer. This is one of the 78 exhibited traditional Chinese medical surgical instruments in the late Qing Dynasty collected by purchasing, solicitation, donation, etc. It is preserved in basically good condition. The point of the hook shows sign of use, while slight rust appears on the hilt.

Preserved in Chinese Medical Association/ Museum of Chinese Medicine, Shanghai University of Traditional Chinese Medicine

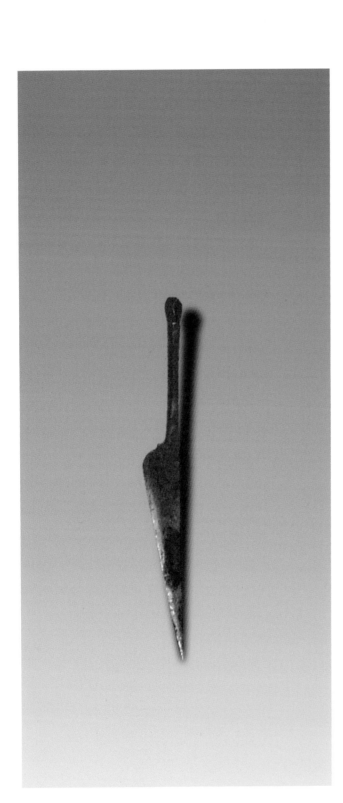

外科斜刃刀

清

铁质

通长 10.5 厘米

柄：宽 0.4 厘米

刃：长 5.9 厘米

Surgical Scalpel with Oblique Blade

Qing Dynasty

Iron

Length 10.5 cm

Hilt: Width 0.4 cm

Blade: Length 5.9 cm

直形，为外科手术用具。斜刃刀是中医外科
最基本的手术用具，主要用做切开疮痈。这
是该馆通过自购、征集、受捐等方式收藏展
出的 78 件清末中医外科手术用具之一。保
存基本完好，钩尖处有使用痕迹，手柄处有
轻微锈斑。

中华医学会 / 上海中医药大学医史博物馆藏

The straight scalpel was used as a surgical
instrument. Surgical scalpels with oblique
blade are the most basic surgical instrument
for incising skin ulcer. This is one of the 78
exhibited traditional Chinese medical surgical
instruments in the late Qing Dynasty collected
by purchasing, solicitation, donation, etc. It is
preserved in basically good condition. The point
of the hook shows sign of use, while slight rust
appears on the hilt.

Preserved in Chinese Medical Association/
Museum of Chinese Medicine, Shanghai
University of Traditional Chinese Medicine

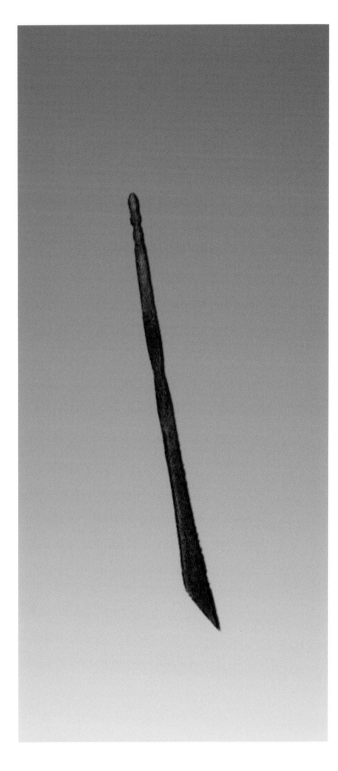

外科斜刃刀

清

铁质

通长 6.9 厘米

柄：宽 0.2 厘米

刃：长 1 厘米

Surgical Scalpel with Oblique Blade

Qing Dynasty

Iron

Length 6.9 cm

Hilt: Width 0.2 cm

Blade: Length 1 cm

直形，为外科手术用具。斜刃刀是中医外科最基本的手术用具，主要用做切开疮痈。这是该馆通过自购、征集、受捐等方式收藏展出的78件清末中医外科手术用具之一。保存基本完好，钩尖处有使用痕迹，手柄处有轻微锈斑。

中华医学会／上海中医药大学医史博物馆藏

The straight scalpel was used as a surgical instrument. Surgical scalpels with oblique blade are the most basic surgical instrument for incising skin ulcer. This is one of the 78 exhibited traditional Chinese medical surgical instruments in the late Qing Dynasty collected by purchasing, solicitation, donation, etc. It is preserved in basically good condition. The point of the hook shows sign of use, while slight rust appears on the hilt.

Preserved in Chinese Medical Association/ Museum of Chinese Medicine, Shanghai University of Traditional Chinese Medicine

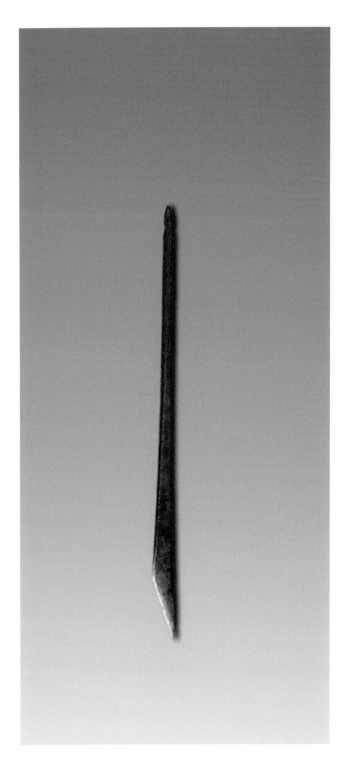

外科斜刃刀

清

铁质

通长 9.5 厘米

柄：宽 0.3 厘米

刃：长 1.6 厘米

Surgical Scalpel with Oblique Blade

Qing Dynasty

Iron

Length 9.5 cm

Hilt: Width 0.3 cm

Blade: Length 1.6 cm

直形，为外科手术用具。斜刃刀是中医外科最基本的手术用具，主要用做切开疮痈。这是该馆通过自购、征集、受捐等方式收藏展出的 78 件清末中医外科手术用具之一。保存基本完好，钩尖处有使用痕迹，手柄处有轻微锈斑。

中华医学会 / 上海中医药大学医史博物馆藏

The straight scalpel was used as a surgical instrument. Surgical scalpels with oblique blade are the most basic surgical instrument for incising skin ulcer. This is one of the 78 exhibited traditional Chinese medical surgical instruments in the late Qing Dynasty collected by purchasing, solicitation, donation, etc. It is preserved in basically good condition. The point of the hook shows sign of use, while slight rust appears on the hilt.

Preserved in Chinese Medical Association/ Museum of Chinese Medicine, Shanghai University of Traditional Chinese Medicine

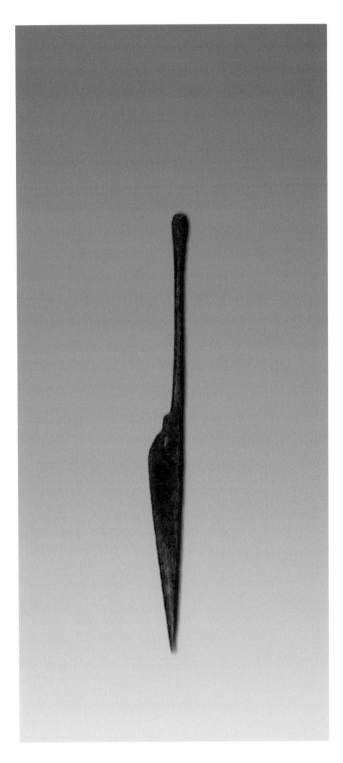

外科斜刃刀

清

铁质

通长 8.1 厘米

柄：宽 0.2 厘米

刃：长 3.7 厘米

Surgical Scalpel with Oblique Blade

Qing Dynasty

Iron

Length 8.1 cm

Hilt: Width 0.2 cm

Blade: Length 3.7 cm

直形，为外科手术用具。斜刃刀是中医外科最基本的手术用具，主要用做切开疮痈。这是该馆通过自购、征集、受捐等方式收藏展出的 78 件清末中医外科手术用具之一。保存基本完好，钩尖处有使用痕迹，手柄处有轻微锈斑。

中华医学会 / 上海中医药大学医史博物馆藏

The straight scalpel was used as a surgical instrument. Surgical scalpels with oblique blade are the most basic surgical instrument for incising skin ulcer. This is one of the 78 exhibited traditional Chinese medical surgical instruments in the late Qing Dynasty collected by purchasing, solicitation, donation, etc. It is preserved in basically good condition. The point of the hook shows sign of use, while slight rust appears on the hilt.

Preserved in Chinese Medical Association/ Museum of Chinese Medicine, Shanghai University of Traditional Chinese Medicine

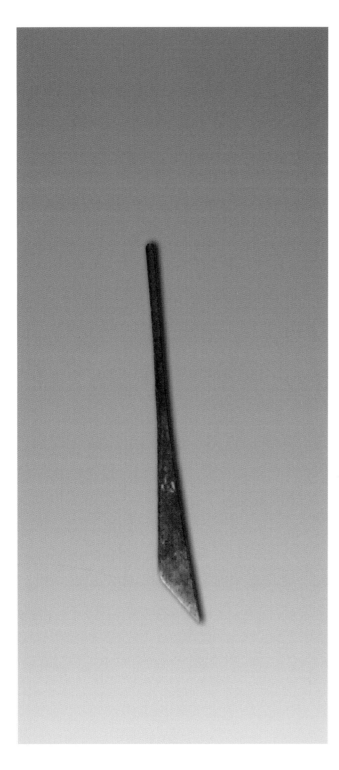

外科斜刃刀

清

铁质

通长 8 厘米

柄：宽 0.3 厘米

刃：长 1.4 厘米

Surgical Scalpel with Oblique Blade

Qing Dynasty

Iron

Length 8 cm

Hilt: Width 0.3 cm

Blade: Length 1.4 cm

直形，为外科手术用具。斜刃刀是中医外科

最基本的手术用具，主要用做切开疮痈。这

是该馆通过自购、征集、受捐等方式收藏展

出的 78 件清末中医外科手术用具之一。保

存基本完好，钩尖处有使用痕迹，手柄处有

轻微锈斑。

中华医学会 / 上海中医药大学医史博物馆藏

The straight scalpel was used as a surgical
instrument. Surgical scalpels with oblique
blade are the most basic surgical instrument
for incising skin ulcer. This is one of the 78
exhibited traditional Chinese medical surgical
instruments in the late Qing Dynasty collected
by purchasing, solicitation, donation, etc. It is
preserved in basically good condition. The point
of the hook shows sign of use, while slight rust
appears on the hilt.

Preserved in Chinese Medical Association/
Museum of Chinese Medicine, Shanghai
University of Traditional Chinese Medicine

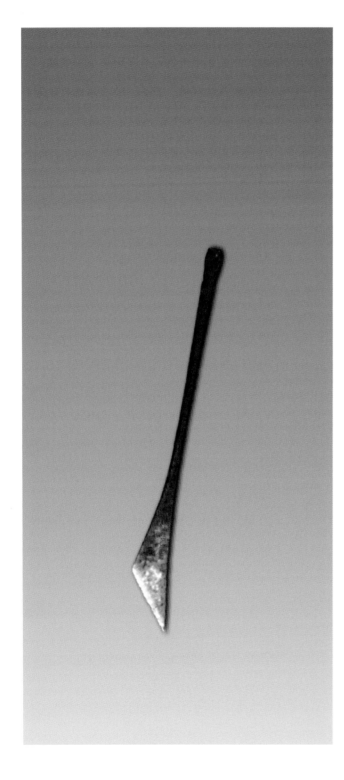

外科斜刃刀

清

铁质

通长 7.7 厘米

柄：宽 0.3 厘米

刃：长 1.5 厘米

Surgical Scalpel with Oblique Blade

Qing Dynasty

Iron

Length 7.7 cm

Hilt: Width 0.3 cm

Blade: Length 1.5 cm

直形，为外科手术用具。斜刃刀是中医外科最基本的手术用具，主要用做切开疮痈。这是该馆通过自购、征集、受捐等方式收藏展出的 78 件清末中医外科手术用具之一。保存基本完好，钩尖处有使用痕迹，手柄处有轻微锈斑。

中华医学会 / 上海中医药大学医史博物馆藏

The straight scalpel was used as a surgical instrument. Surgical scalpels with oblique blade are the most basic surgical instrument for incising skin ulcer. This is one of the 78 exhibited traditional Chinese medical surgical instruments in the late Qing Dynasty collected by purchasing, solicitation, donation, etc. It is preserved in basically good condition. The point of the hook shows sign of use, while slight rust appears on the hilt.

Preserved in Chinese Medical Association/ Museum of Chinese Medicine, Shanghai University of Traditional Chinese Medicine

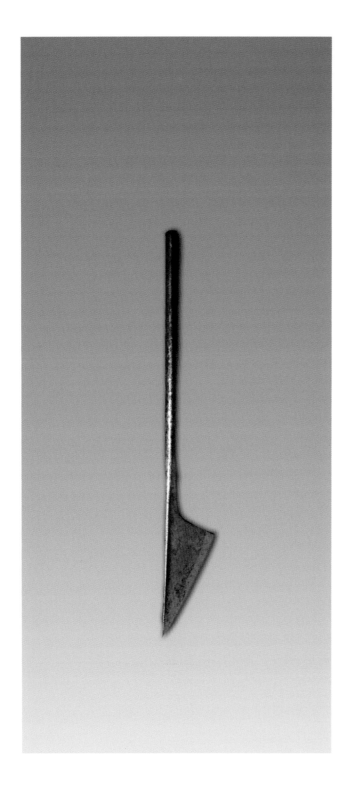

外科斜刃刀

清

铁质

通长 13 厘米

柄：径 0.4 厘米

刃：长 3.82 厘米

Surgical Scalpel with Oblique Blade

Qing Dynasty

Iron

Length 13 cm

Hilt: Diameter 0.4 cm

Blade: Length 3.82 cm

直形，为外科手术用具。斜刃刀是中医外科
最基本的手术用具，主要用做切开疮痈。这
是该馆接受卢大均中医师捐献而收藏的一组
清末中医外科手术用具之一。保存基本完好，
钩尖处有使用痕迹，手柄处有轻微锈斑。

中华医学会 / 上海中医药大学医史博物馆藏

The straight scalpel was used as a surgical
instrument. Surgical scalpels with oblique
blade are the most basic surgical instrument for
incising skin ulcer. This is one of a series of
traditional Chinese medical surgical instruments
in the late Qing Dynasty donated by practitioner
Lu Dajun of traditional Chinese medicine. It is
preserved in basically good condition. The point
of the hook shows sign of use, while slight rust
appears on the hilt.

Preserved in Chinese Medical Association/
Museum of Chinese Medicine, Shanghai
University of Traditional Chinese Medicine

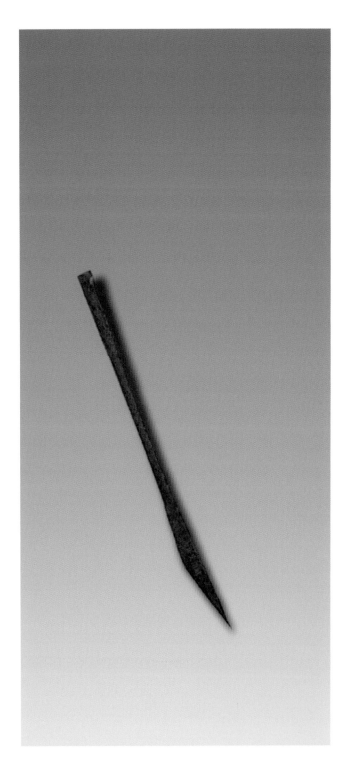

外科斜刃刀

清

铁质

通长 6.8 厘米

柄：宽 0.2 厘米

刃：长 1.2 厘米

Surgical Scalpel with Oblique Edge

Qing Dynasty

Iron

Length 6.8 cm

Hilt: Width 0.2 cm

Blade: Length 1.2 cm

直形，为外科手术用具。斜刃刀是中医外科最基本的手术用具，主要用做切开疮痈。这是该馆通过自购、征集、受捐等方式收藏展出的78件清末中医外科手术用具之一。保存基本完好，钩尖处有使用痕迹，手柄处有轻微锈斑。

中华医学会 / 上海中医药大学医史博物馆藏

The straight scalpel was used as a surgical instrument. Surgical scalpels with oblique blade are the most basic surgical instrument for incising skin ulcer. This is one of the 78 exhibited traditional Chinese medical surgical instruments in the late Qing Dynasty collected by purchasing, solicitation, donation, etc. It is preserved in basically good condition. The point of the hook shows sign of use, while slight rust appears on the hilt.

Preserved in Chinese Medical Association/ Museum of Chinese Medicine, Shanghai University of Traditional Chinese Medicine

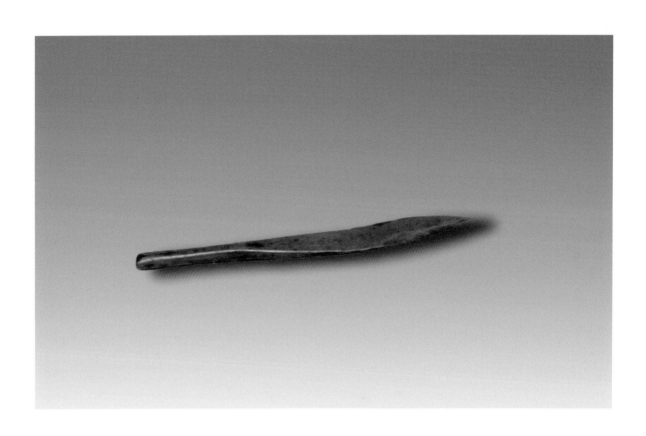

柳叶刀

清

铜质

长 6 厘米，宽 0.6 厘米

Lancet (Liu Ye Dao)

Qing Dynasty

Copper

Length 6 cm/ Width 0.6 cm

刃部呈弧形，刀身形似柳叶，故得名。柳叶刀是外科重要的手术器械，适合切开浅层较长切口。由民间征集。

成都中医药大学中医药传统文化博物馆藏

The edge slightly bent, the lancet got its Chinese name Liu Ye Dao from the salix leaf-shaped body. This knife is an important surgical appliance in surgical operation, which is fit to cut the superficial and long incisions. It was collected by a non-governmental organization.

Preserved in Museum of Traditional Chinese Medicine Culture, Chengdu University of Traditional Chinese Medicine

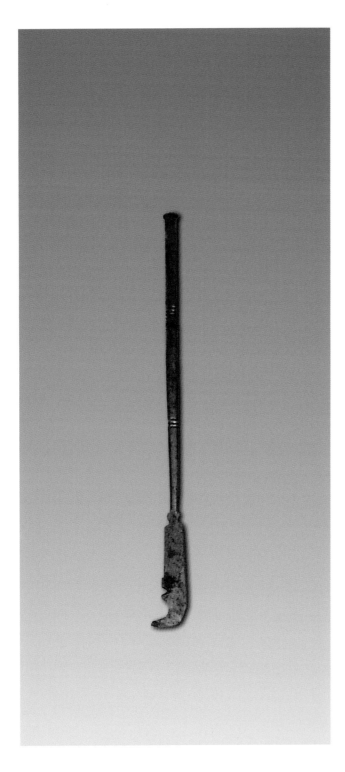

外科弯刃刀

清

铁质

通长 12.5 厘米

刃：长 3 厘米，宽 1 厘米

柄：宽 0.4 厘米

Surgical Knife with Curving Edge

Qing Dynasty

Iron

Length 12.5 cm

Blade: Length 3 cm/ Width 1 cm

Hilt: Width 0.4 cm

长戟形，为外科手术用具。这是该馆通过自购、征集、受捐等方式收藏展出的 78 件清末中医外科手术用具之一。《外科心法真验指掌》中陈述的弯刃刀有内弯式和外弯式两种，前者"为取皮里暗处溃肉，可以弯割去之"；后者"外刃必滑锋，为去皮里深处腐肉，可以易割取之"。此件为外弯式戟形弯刃刀。保存基本完好，钩尖处有使用痕迹，手柄处有轻微锈斑。

中华医学会 / 上海中医药大学医史博物馆藏

This halberd-like knife is a tool for surgical operations. This is one of the 78 surgical appliances in traditional Chinese medicine surgery of the late Qing Dynasty which were displayed in this museum. According to the record of *Wai Ke Xin Fa Zhen Yan Zhi Zhang* (a medical book on surgery), there are inner edge and outer edge knives. The former "can be used for cutting out the ulcerated flesh hidden in the skin", while the latter "must be smooth and sharp to cut out the flesh from inside of the skin". It is a halberd-like knife with an outer edge. This knife is basically well-preserved. There are some signs of use on the crook and tip, with slight rust spots covered on the handle.

Preserved in Chinese Medical Association/Museum of Chinese Medicine, Shanghai University of Traditional Chinese Medicine

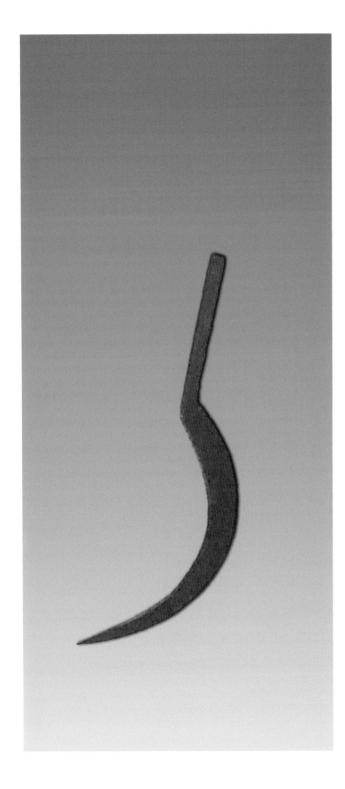

外科弯刃刀

清

铁质

刃：长 6.3 厘米，宽 0.6 厘米

柄：长 3 厘米，宽 0.3 厘米

Surgical Knife with Curving Edge

Qing Dynasty

Iron

Blade: Length 6.3 cm/ Width 0.6 cm

Hilt: Length 3 cm/ Width 0.3 cm

弯镰形，为外科手术用具。这是该馆通过自购、征集、受捐等方式收藏展出的78件清末中医外科手术用具之一。《外科心法真验指掌》中陈述的弯刃刀有内弯式和外弯式两种。前者"为取皮里暗处溃肉，可以弯割去之"，后者"外刃必滑锋，为去皮里深处腐肉，可以易割取之"。此件为内弯式弯刃刀。保存基本完好，钩尖处有使用痕迹，手柄处有轻微锈斑。

中华医学会 / 上海中医药大学医史博物馆藏

This curved sickle-like knife is a tool for surgical operations. This is one of the 78 surgical appliances in traditional Chinese medicine surgery of the late Qing Dynasty which were displayed in this museum. According to the record of *Wai Ke Xin Fa Zhen Yan Zhi Zhang* (a medical book on surgery), there are inner edge and outer edge knives. The former "can be used for cutting out the ulcerated flesh hidden in the skin", while the latter "must be smooth and sharp to cut out the flesh from inside of the skin". It is a knife with incurved edge. This knife is basically well-preserved. There are some signs of use on the crook and tip, with slight rust spots covered on the handle.

Preserved in Chinese Medical Association/Museum of Chinese Medicine, Shanghai University of Traditional Chinese Medicine

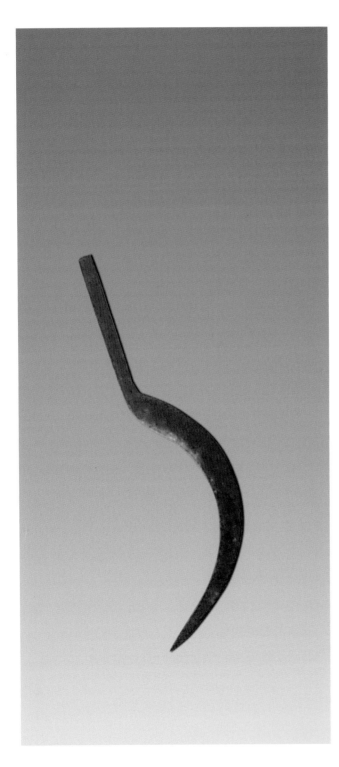

外科弯刃刀

清

铁质

刃：长 6.5 厘米，宽 0.7 厘米

柄：长 2.9 厘米，宽 0.3 厘米

Surgical Knife with Curving Edge

Qing Dynasty

Iron

Blade: Length 6.5 cm/ Width 0.7 cm

Hilt: Length 2.9 cm/ Width 0.3 cm

弯镰形，为外科手术用具。这是该馆通过自购、征集、受捐等方式收藏展出的 78 件清末中医外科手术用具之一。《外科心法真验指掌》中陈述的弯刃刀有内弯式和外弯式两种，前者"为取皮里暗处溃肉，可以弯割去之"；后者"外刃必滑锋，为去皮里深处腐肉，可以易割取之"。此件为内弯式弯刃刀。保存基本完好，钩尖处有使用痕迹，手柄处有轻微锈斑。

中华医学会 / 上海中医药大学医史博物馆藏

This curved sickle-like knife is a tool for surgical operations. This is one of the 78 surgical appliances in traditional Chinese medicine surgery of the late Qing Dynasty which were displayed in this museum. According to the record of *Wai Ke Xin Fa Zhen Yan Zhi Zhang* (a medical book on surgery), there are inner edge and outer edge knives. The former "can be used for cutting out the ulcerated flesh hidden in the skin", while the latter "must be smooth and sharp to cut out the carrion from inside of the skin". It is a knife with incurved edge. This knife is basically well-preserved. There are some signs of use on the crook and tip, with slight rust spots covered on the handle.

Preserved in Chinese Medical Association/Museum of Chinese Medicine, Shanghai University of Traditional Chinese Medicine

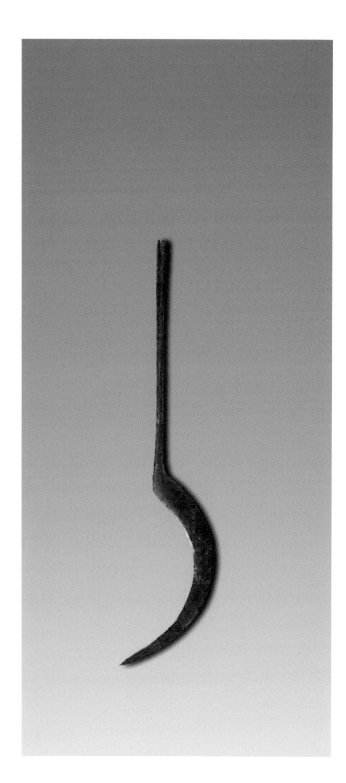

外科弯刃刀

清

铁质

刃：长 6.3 厘米，宽 0.7 厘米

柄：长 6.2 厘米，宽 0.3 厘米

Surgical Knife with Curving Edge

Qing Dynasty

Iron

Blade: Length 6.3 cm/ Width 0.7 cm

Hilt: Length 6.2 cm/ Width 0.3 cm

弯镰形，为外科手术用具。这是该馆通过自购、征集、受捐等方式收藏展出的 78 件清末中医外科手术用具之一。《外科心法真验指掌》中陈述的弯刃刀有内弯式和外弯式两种。前者"为取皮里暗处溃肉，可以弯割去之"；后者"外刃必滑锋，为去皮里深处腐肉，可以易割取之"。此件为内弯式弯刃刀。保存基本完好，钩尖处有使用痕迹，手柄处有轻微锈斑。

中华医学会 / 上海中医药大学医史博物馆藏

This curved sickle-like knife is a tool for surgical operations. This is one of the 78 surgical appliances in traditional Chinese medicine surgery of the late Qing Dynasty which were displayed in this museum. According to the record of *Wai Ke Xin Fa Zhen Yan Zhi Zhang* (a medical book on surgery), there are inner edge and outer edge knives. The former "can be used for cutting out the ulcerated flesh hidden in the skin", while the latter "must be smooth and sharp to cut out the flesh from inside of the skin". It is a knife with incurved edge. This knife is basically well-preserved. There are some signs of use on the crook and tip, with slight rust spots covered on the handle.

Preserved in Chinese Medical Association/Museum of Chinese Medicine, Shanghai University of Traditional Chinese Medicine

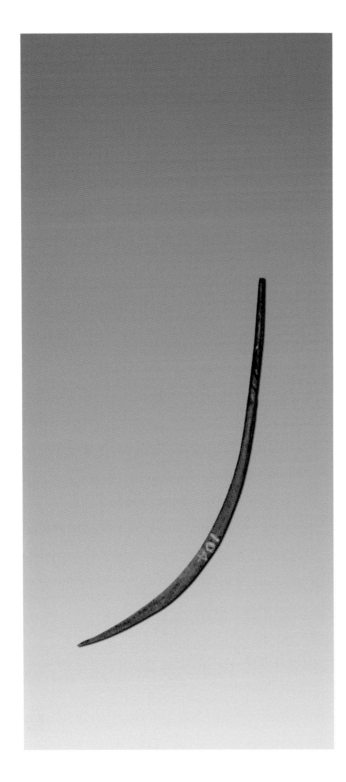

外科弯刃刀

清

铜质

刃：长 5.3 厘米，宽 0.4 厘米

Surgical Knife with Curving Edge

Qing Dynasty

Copper

Blade: Length 5.3 cm/ Width 0.4 cm

长柳叶形，为外科手术用具。这是该馆通过自购、征集、受捐等方式收藏展出的78件清末中医外科手术用具之一。《外科心法真验指掌》中陈述的弯刃刀有内弯式和外弯式两种，前者"为取皮里暗处溃肉，可以弯割去之"；后者"外刃必滑锋，为去皮里深处腐肉，可以易割取之"。此件为内弯式弯刃刀。保存基本完好，钩尖处有使用痕迹，手柄处可见轻微锈斑。

中华医学会 / 上海中医药大学医史博物馆藏

This long salix leaf-shaped knife is a tool for surgical operations. This is one of the 78 surgical appliances in traditional Chinese medicine surgery of the late Qing Dynasty which were displayed in this museum. According to the record of *Wai Ke Xin Fa Zhen Yan Zhi Zhang* (a medical book on surgery), there are inner edge and outer edge knives. The former "can be used for cutting out the ulcerated flesh hidden in the skin", while the latter "must be smooth and sharp to cut out the flesh from inside of the skin". It is a knife with incurved edge. This knife is basically well-preserved. There are some signs of use on the crook and tip, with slight rust spots covered on the handle.

Preserved in Chinese Medical Association/Museum of Chinese Medicine, Shanghai University of Traditional Chinese Medicine

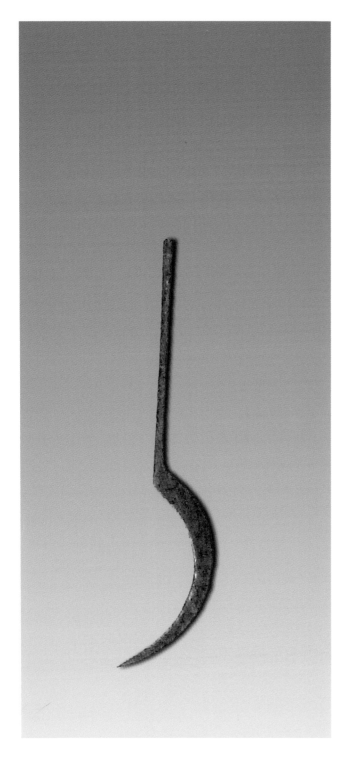

外科弯刃刀

清

铁质

刃：长 6.5 厘米，宽 0.7 厘米

柄：长 6.1 厘米，宽 0.3 厘米

Surgical Knife with Curving Edge

Qing Dynasty

Iron

Blade: Length 6.5 cm/ Width 0.7 cm

Hilt: Length 6.1 cm/ Width 0.3 cm

弯镰形，为外科手术用具。这是该馆通过自购、征集、受捐等方式收藏展出的 78 件清末中医外科手术用具之一。《外科心法真验指掌》中陈述的弯刃刀有内弯式和外弯式两种，前者"为取皮里暗处溃肉，可以弯割去之"；后者"外刃必滑锋，为去皮里深处腐肉，可以易割取之"。此件为内弯式弯刃刀。保存基本完好，钩尖处有使用痕迹，手柄处可见轻微锈斑。

中华医学会 / 上海中医药大学医史博物馆藏

This curved sickle-like knife is a tool for surgical operations. This is one of the 78 surgical appliances in traditional Chinese medicine surgery of the late Qing Dynasty which were displayed in this museum. According to the record of *Wai Ke Xin Fa Zhen Yan Zhi Zhang* (a medical book on surgery), there are inner edge and outer edge knives. The former "can be used for cutting out the ulcerated flesh hidden in the skin", while the latter "must be smooth and sharp to cut out the flesh from inside of the skin". It is a knife with incurved edge. This knife is basically well-preserved. There are some signs of use on the crook and tip, with slight rust spots covered on the handle.

Preserved in Chinese Medical Association/Museum of Chinese Medicine, Shanghai University of Traditional Chinese Medicine

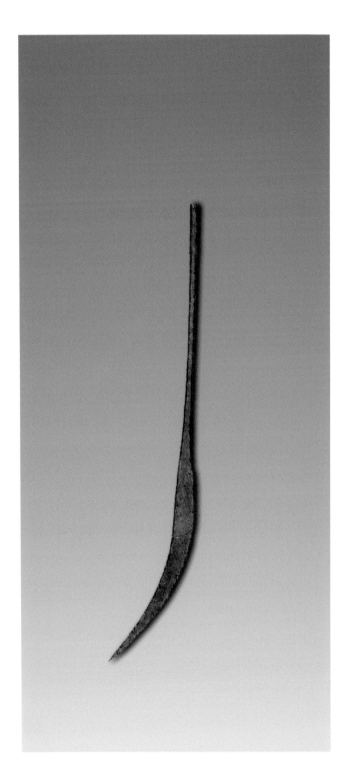

外科弯刃刀

清

铁质

刃：长 5.3 厘米，宽 0.4 厘米

Surgical Knife with Curving Edge

Qing Dynasty

Iron

Blade: Length 5.3 cm/ Width 0.4 cm

长柳叶形，为外科手术用具。这是该馆通过自购、征集、受捐等方式收藏展出的78件清末中医外科手术用具之一。《外科心法真验指掌》中陈述的弯刃刀有内弯式和外弯式两种，前者"为取皮里暗处溃肉，可以弯割去之"；后者"外刃必滑锋，为去皮里深处腐肉，可以易割取之"。此件为内弯式弯刃刀。保存基本完好，钩尖处有使用痕迹，手柄处有轻微锈斑。

中华医学会 / 上海中医药大学医史博物馆藏

This long salix leaf-shaped knife is a tool for surgical operations. This is one of the 78 surgical appliances in traditional Chinese medicine surgery of the late Qing Dynasty which were displayed in this museum. According to the record of *Wai Ke Xin Fa Zhen Yan Zhi Zhang* (a medical book on surgery), there are inner edge and outer edge knives. The former "can be used for cutting out the ulcerated flesh hidden in the skin", while the latter "must be smooth and sharp to cut out the flesh from inside of the skin". It is a knife with incurved edge. This knife is basically well-preserved. There are some signs of use on the crook and tip, with slight rust spots covered on the handle.

Preserved in Chinese Medical Association/Museum of Chinese Medicine, Shanghai University of Traditional Chinese Medicine

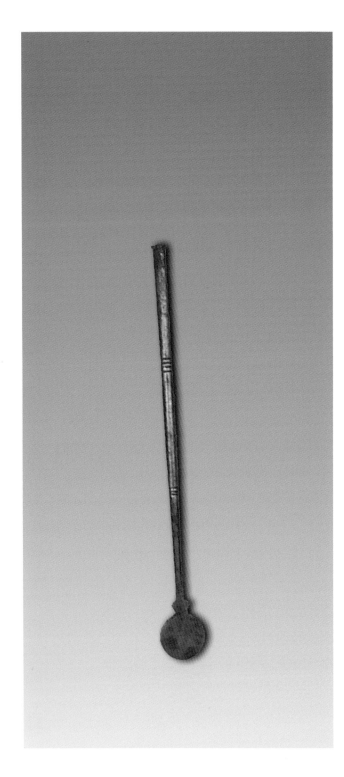

外科圆刃铲刀

清

铁质

通长 12 厘米

柄：径 0.4 厘米

铲部：宽 1.3 厘米

Surgical Scraper Knife with Round Edge

Qing Dynasty

Iron

Length 12 cm

Hilt: Diameter 0.4 cm

Scraper: Width 1.3 cm

长铲形，为外科常用手术用具。此铲之铲部呈圆饼状，圆柄上部有旋纹。《外科明隐集》称这种铲刀"用其割除深陷之内瘀腐"，亦做"割除死腐余皮"之用。这是该馆通过自购、征集、受捐等方式收藏展出的78件清末中医外科手术用具之一。保存基本完好，刃部有使用痕迹，铲身可见有轻微锈斑。

中华医学会/上海中医药大学医史博物馆藏

This long scraper-like knife is a tool for surgical operations. The shovel part of this scraper is like a round cake, and the cylinder handle is decorated with vortex patterns. According to the book *Wai Ke Ming Yin Ji* (a medical book on surgery), this kind of scraper knife was used to cut the slough deep inside or on the rotten skin. This is one of the 78 surgical appliances in traditional Chinese medicine surgery of the late Qing Dynasty which were displayed in this museum and collected by purchasing, solicitation and donation and so on. It is basically well-preserved. There are some signs of use on the edge, with slight rust spots covered on the body of scraper.

Preserved in Chinese Medical Association/Museum of Chinese Medicine, Shanghai University of Traditional Chinese Medicine

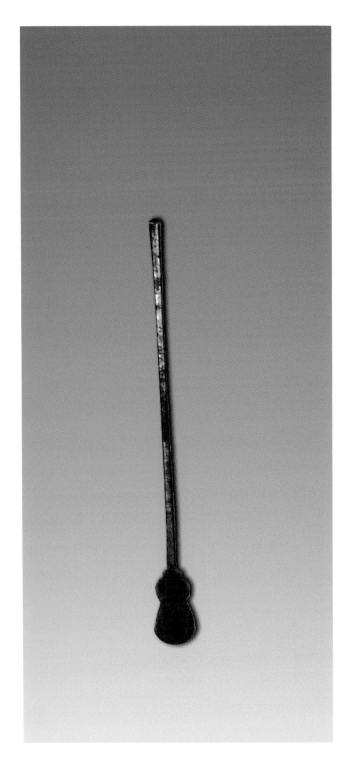

外科圆刃铲刀

清

铁质

通长 12.1 厘米

柄：径 0.3 厘米

铲部：宽 1.2 厘米

Surgical Scraper Knife with Round Edge

Qing Dynasty

Iron

Length 12.1 cm

Hilt: Diameter 0.3 cm

Scraper: Width 1.2 cm

长铲形，为外科常用手术用具。此铲之铲部呈琵琶状，圆柄上部有旋纹。《外科明隐集》称这种铲刀"用其割除深陷之内瘀腐"，亦做"割除死腐余皮"之用。这是该馆通过自购、征集、受捐等方式收藏展出的 78 件清末中医外科手术用具之一。保存基本完好，刃部有使用痕迹，铲身可见有轻微锈斑。

中华医学会 / 上海中医药大学医史博物馆藏

This long scraper-like knife is a tool for surgical operations. The shovel part of this scraper is like a Chinese lute, and the cylinder handle is decorated with vortex patterns. According to the book *Wai Ke Ming Yin Ji* (a medical book on surgery), this kind of scraper knife was used to cut the slough deep inside or on the rotten skin. This is one of the 78 surgical appliances in traditional Chinese medicine surgery of the late Qing Dynasty which were displayed in this museum and collected by purchasing, solicitation and donation and so on. It is basically well-preserved. There are some signs of use on the edge, with slight rust spots covered on the body of scraper.

Preserved in Chinese Medical Association/Museum of Chinese Medicine, Shanghai University of Traditional Chinese Medicine

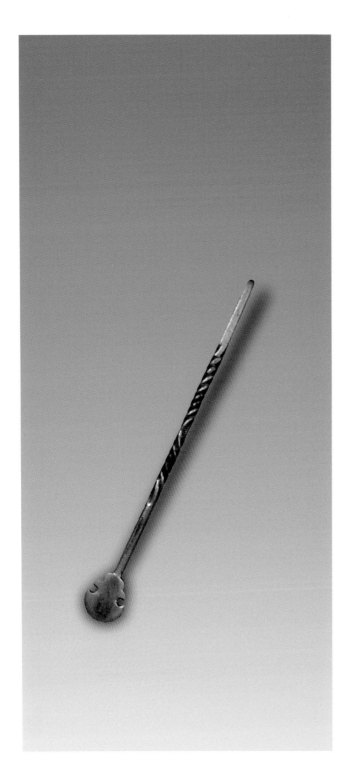

外科圆刃铲刀

清

铜质

通长 11.7 厘米

柄：径 0.3 厘米

铲部：宽 1.4 厘米

Surgical Scraper Knife with Round Edge

Qing Dynasty

Copper

Length 11.7 cm

Hilt: Diameter 0.3 cm

Scraper: Width 1.4 cm

长铲形，为常用外科手术用具。此铲之铲部呈圆饼状，饼状铲头两侧各有一小豁口，圆柄有旋纹。《外科明隐集》称这种铲刀"用其割除深陷之内瘀腐"，亦做"割除死腐余皮"之用。这是该馆通过自购、征集、受捐等方式收藏展出的78件清末中医外科手术用具之一。保存基本完好，刃部有使用痕迹，铲身可见有轻微锈斑。

中华医学会/上海中医药大学医史博物馆藏

This long scraper-like knife is a tool for surgical operations. The shovel part of this scraper is like a round cake, and both sides of the cake-shaped head have a small breach. The round handle is decorated with vortex patterns. According to the book *Wai Ke Ming Yin Ji* (a medical book on surgery), this kind of scraper knife was used to cut the slough deep inside or on the rotten skin. This is one of the 78 surgical appliances in traditional Chinese medicine surgery of the late Qing Dynasty which were displayed in this museum and collected by purchasing, solicitation and donation and so on. It is basically well-preserved. There are some signs of use on the edge, with slight rust spots covered on the body of scraper.

Preserved in Chinese Medical Association/Museum of Chinese Medicine, Shanghai University of Traditional Chinese Medicine

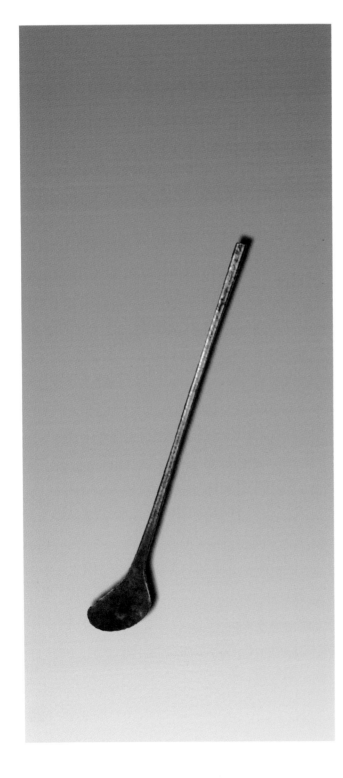

外科圆刃铲刀

清

铁质

通长 11.8 厘米

柄：径 0.3 厘米

铲部：宽 1.4 厘米

Surgical Scraper Knife with Round Edge

Qing Dynasty

Iron

Length 11.8 cm

Hilt: Diameter 0.3 cm

Scraper: Width 1.4 cm

长铲形，为常用外科手术用具。此铲之铲部呈扁圆状，圆柄倾斜，上部有旋纹。《外科明隐集》称这种铲刀"用其割除深陷之内瘀腐"，亦做"割除死腐余皮"之用。这是该馆通过自购、征集、受捐等方式收藏展出的 78 件清末中医外科手术用具之一。保存基本完好，刃部有使用痕迹，铲身可见有轻微锈斑。

中华医学会 / 上海中医药大学医史博物馆藏

This long scraper-like knife is a tool for surgical operations. The shovel part of this scraper is flattened round shape, and the cylinder handle is oblique, with the design of vortex patterns on its upper part. According to the book *Wai Ke Ming Yin Ji* (a medical book on surgery), this kind of scraper knife was used to cut the slough deep inside or on the rotten skin. This is one of the 78 surgical appliances in traditional Chinese medicine surgery of the late Qing Dynasty which were displayed in this museum and collected by purchasing, solicitation and donation and so on. It is basically well-preserved. There are some signs of use on the edge, with slight rust spots covered on the body of scraper. Preserved in Chinese Medical Association/Museum of Chinese Medicine, Shanghai University of Traditional Chinese Medicine

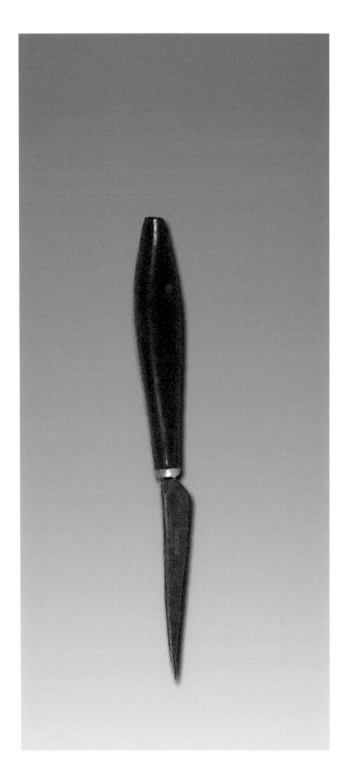

外科尖刀

清

铁质木柄

通长 9.1 厘米

刀：长 4 厘米

刃：长 3.6 厘米，宽 0.7 厘米

Surgical Sharp Knife

Qing Dynasty

Iron, Wooden Handle

Length 9.1 cm

Knife: Length 4 cm

Blade: Length 3.6 cm/ Width 0.7 cm

匕首形，为外科手术用具。此尖刀为木柄单刃铁刀，刃口长而锋利，便于着力握持以切入肌肤，是清末中医外科常用刀具。这是该馆通过自购、征集、受捐等方式收藏展出的78件清末中医外科手术用具之一。保存基本完好，刃部有使用痕迹，刀身可见有轻微锈斑。

中华医学会 / 上海中医药大学医史博物馆藏

This dagger-like knife is a tool for surgical operations. This sharp knife belongs to the single-edged iron knife with a wodden handle, and the cutting edge is long and sharp in order to cut into the skin by putting force on it. It was commonly used in the late Qing Dynasty. This is one of the 78 surgical appliances in traditional Chinese medicine surgery of the late Qing Dynasty which were displayed in this museum and collected by purchasing, solicitation, donation and so on. It is basically well-preserved. There are some signs of use on the edge, with slight rust spots covered on the body of knife.

Preserved in Chinese Medical Association/ Museum of Chinese Medicine, Shanghai University of Traditional Chinese Medicine

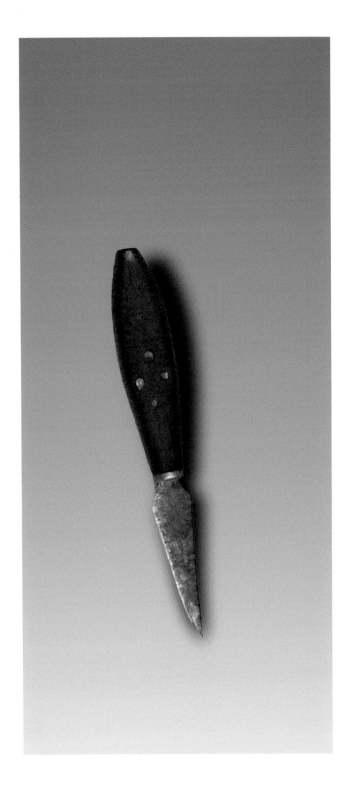

外科尖刀

清

铁质木柄

通长 9.2 厘米

刀：长 3.8 厘米

刃：长 3.4 厘米，宽 1 厘米

Surgical Sharp Knife

Qing Dynasty

Iron, Wooden Handle

Length 9.2 cm

Knife: Length 3.8 cm

Blade: Length 3.4 cm/ Width 1 cm

匕首形，为外科手术用具。此尖刀为木柄单
刃铁刀，刃口长而锋利，便于着力握持以切
入肌肤，是清末中医外科常用刀具。这是该
馆通过自购、征集、受捐等方式收藏展出的
78 件清末中医外科手术用具之一。保存基本
完好，刃部有使用痕迹，刀身可见有轻微锈斑。

中华医学会 / 上海中医药大学医史博物馆藏

This dagger-like knife is a tool for surgical
operations. This sharp knife belongs to the
single-edged iron knife with a wodden handle,
and the cutting edge is long and sharp in order
to cut into the skin by putting force on it. It
was commonly used in the late Qing Dynasty.
This is one of the 78 surgical appliances in
traditional Chinese medicine surgery of the
late Qing Dynasty which were displayed in
this museum and collected by purchasing,
solicitation, donation and so on. It is basically
well-preserved. There are some signs of use on
the edge, with slight rust spots covered on the
body of knife.

Preserved in Chinese Medical Association/
Museum of Chinese Medicine, Shanghai
University of Traditional Chinese Medicine

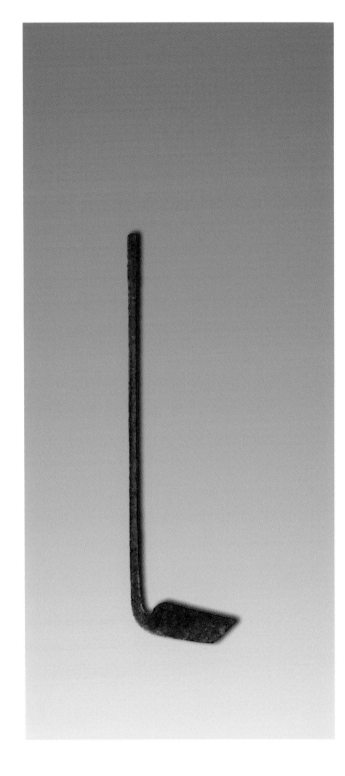

外科钩镰刀

清

铁质

通长 8.5 厘米

刃：长 1.6 厘米，宽 0.7 厘米

柄：宽 0.2 厘米

Surgical Sickle-like Knife with Hook

Qing Dynasty

Iron

Length 8.5 cm

Blade: Length 1.6 cm/ Width 0.7 cm

Hilt: Width 0.2 cm

镰刀形，为外科手术用具。《外科心法真验
指掌》载："此镰遇疮有粘脓不断，以镊捏
住，用镰割之。"这是该馆通过自购、征集、
受捐等方式收藏展出的 78 件清末中医外科
手术用具之一。保存基本完好，钩尖处有使
用痕迹，手柄处有轻微锈斑。

中华医学会 / 上海中医药大学医史博物馆藏

This sickle-like knife is a tool for surgical
operations. According to the book of surgery,
Wai Ke Xin Fa Zhen Yan Zhi Zhang, this
sickle-like knife can be used for cutting out
the ulcerated flesh with viscous pus pinched
by a tweezer. This is one of the 78 surgical
appliances in traditional Chinese medicine
surgery of the late Qing Dynasty which were
displayed in this museum and collected by
purchasing, solicitation, donation and so on.
It is basically well-preserved. There are some
signs of use on the crook and tip, with some
rust spots slightly covered on the handle.
Preserved in Chinese Medical Association/
Museum of Chinese Medicine, Shanghai
University of Traditional Chinese Medicine

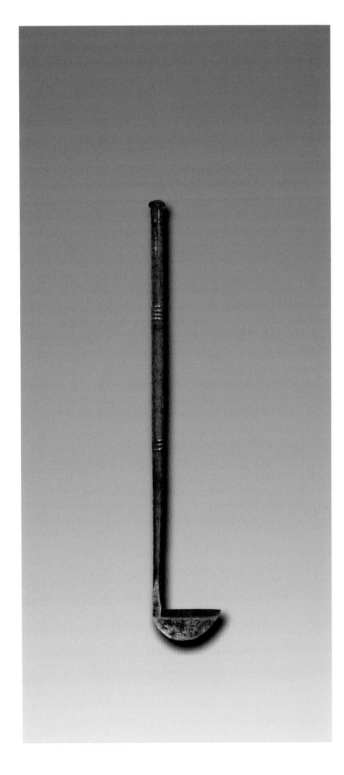

外科钩镰刀

清

铁质

通长 11.8 厘米

刃：长 1.6 厘米，宽 0.8 厘米

柄：宽 0.4 厘米

Surgical Sickle-like Knife with Hook

Qing Dynasty

Iron

Length 11.8 cm

Blade: Length 1.6 cm/ Width 0.8 cm

Hilt: Width 0.4 cm

镰刀形，为外科手术用具。《外科心法真验指掌》载："此镰遇疮有粘脓不断，以镊捏住，用镰割之。"这是该馆通过自购、征集、受捐等方式收藏展出的78件清末中医外科手术用具之一。保存基本完好，钩尖处有使用痕迹，手柄处有轻微锈斑。

中华医学会/上海中医药大学医史博物馆藏

This sickle-like knife is a tool for surgical operations. According to the book of surgery, *Wai Ke Xin Fa Zhen Yan Zhi Zhang*, this sickle-like knife can be used for cutting out the ulcerated flesh with viscous pus pinched by a tweezer. This is one of the 78 surgical appliances in traditional Chinese medicine surgery of the late Qing Dynasty which were displayed in this museum and collected by purchasing, solicitation, donation and so on. It is basically well-preserved. There are some signs of use on the crook and tip, with some rust spots slightly covered on the handle.

Preserved in Chinese Medical Association/ Museum of Chinese Medicine, Shanghai University of Traditional Chinese Medicine

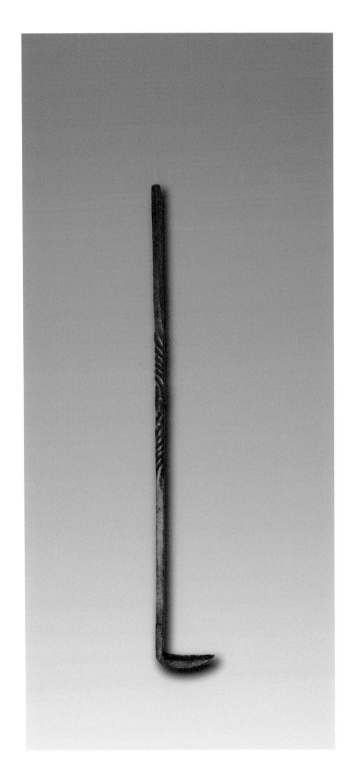

外科钩镰刀

清

铜质

通长 14 厘米

刃：长 2.6 厘米，宽 0.4 厘米

柄：宽 0.3 厘米

Surgical Sickle-like Knife with Hook

Qing Dynasty

Copper

Length 14 cm

Blade: Length 2.6 cm/ Width 0.4 cm

Hilt: Width 0.3 cm

镰刀形，为外科手术用具。《外科心法真验指掌》载："此镰遇疮有粘脓不断，以镊捏住，用镰割之。" 这是该馆通过自购、征集、受捐等方式收藏展出的 78 件清末中医外科手术用具之一。保存基本完好，钩尖处有使用痕迹，手柄处有轻微锈斑。

中华医学会 / 上海中医药大学医史博物馆藏

This sickle-like knife is a tool for surgical operations. According to the book of surgery, *Wai Ke Xin Fa Zhen Yan Zhi Zhang*, this sickle-like knife can be used for cutting out the ulcerated flesh with viscous pus pinched by a tweezer. This is one of the 78 surgical appliances in traditional Chinese medicine surgery of the late Qing Dynasty which were displayed in this museum and collected by purchasing, solicitation, donation and so on. It is basically well-preserved. There are some signs of use on the crook and tip, with some rust spots slightly covered on the handle.
Preserved in Chinese Medical Association/ Museum of Chinese Medicine, Shanghai University of Traditional Chinese Medicine

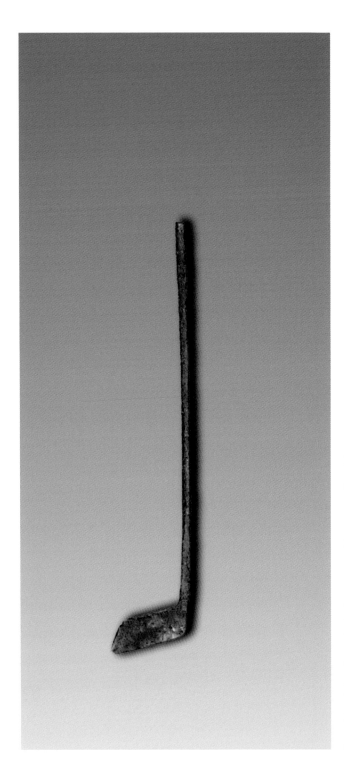

外科钩镰刀

清

铁质

刃：长 6.5 厘米，宽 0.7 厘米

柄：长 6.1 厘米，宽 0.3 厘米

Surgical Sickle-like Knife with Hook

Qing Dynasty

Iron

Blade: Length 6.5 cm/ Width 0.7 cm

Hilt: Length 6.1 cm/ Width 0.3 cm

镰刀形，为外科手术用具。《外科心法真验指掌》载："此镰遇疮有粘脓不断，以镊捏住，用镰割之。"这是该馆通过自购、征集、受捐等方式收藏展出的 78 件清末中医外科手术用具之一。保存基本完好，钩尖处有使用痕迹，手柄处有轻微锈斑。

中华医学会 / 上海中医药大学医史博物馆藏

This sickle-like knife is a tool for surgical operations. According to the book of surgery, *Wai Ke Xin Fa Zhen Yan Zhi Zhang*, this sickle-like knife can be used for cutting out the ulcerated flesh with viscous pus pinched by a tweezer. This is one of the 78 surgical appliances in traditional Chinese medicine surgery of the late Qing Dynasty which were displayed in this museum and collected by purchasing, solicitation, donation and so on. It is basically well-preserved. There are some signs of use on the crook and tip, with some rust spots slightly covered on the handle.

Preserved in Chinese Medical Association/ Museum of Chinese Medicine, Shanghai University of Traditional Chinese Medicine

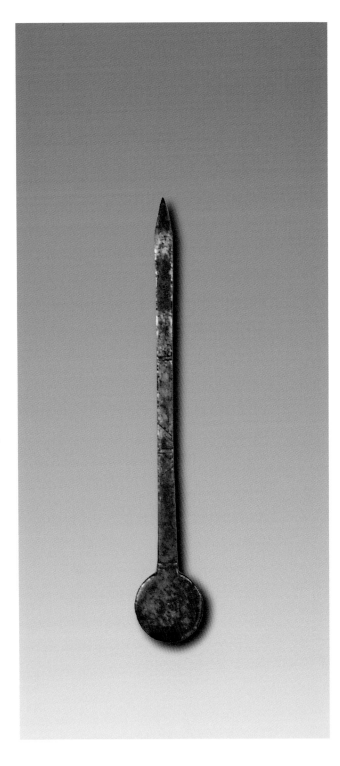

外科两用器

清

铁质

通长 14.8 厘米

柄：径 0.6 厘米

铲部：宽 2.4 厘米

Surgical Appliance of Two-Purpose

Qing Dynasty

Iron

Length 14.8 cm

Hilt: Diameter 0.6 cm

Scraper: Width 2.4 cm

长铲形，为常用外科手术用具。此器一端为锥，另一端呈圆饼状，扁平状长柄。这种用具一端用做锥，另一端可能用来分离肌肉等。这是该馆通过自购、征集、受捐等方式收藏展出的 78 件清末中医外科手术用具之一。保存基本完好，尖部有使用痕迹，器身可见有轻微锈斑。

中华医学会 / 上海中医药大学医史博物馆藏

This long scraper-like knife is a tool for surgical operations. There is an awl at one end of this appliance. The other end is shaped like a round cake, connected by a long tabular-shaped handle. One end was used for boring skin, the other for separating muscles, etc. This is one of the 78 surgical appliances in traditional Chinese medicine surgery of the late Qing Dynasty which were displayed in this museum and collected by purchasing, solicitation, donation and so on. It is basically well-preserved. There are some signs of use on the tip, with some rust spots slightly covered on the body.

Preserved in Chinese Medical Association/ Museum of Chinese Medicine, Shanghai University of Traditional Chinese Medicine

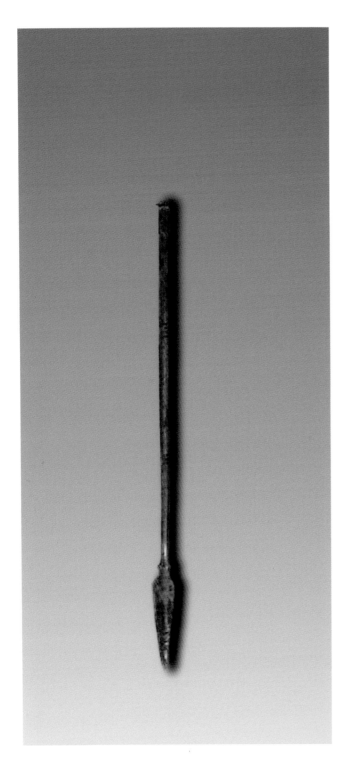

外科簇尖刺锥

清

铁质

通长 11.1 厘米

刃：长 2.5 厘米，宽 0.7 厘米

柄：宽 0.7 厘米

Surgical Awl with Pointed Tip

Qing Dynasty

Iron

Length 11.1 cm

Blade: Length 2.5 cm/ Width 0.7 cm

Hilt: Width 0.7 cm

长锥形，为外科手术用具。此锥为双刃，《喉科心法》称"剑针"，用做"备通脓管之用，取其迅速，痰包亦用此破"。这是该馆通过自购、征集、受捐等方式收藏展出的78件清末中医外科手术用具之一。保存基本完好，刃部有使用痕迹，刀身可见有轻微锈斑。

中华医学会 / 上海中医药大学医史博物馆藏

This long awl-like knife is a tool for surgical operations. This awl has two edges. In the book *Hou Ke Xin Fa* (a medical book on laryngology), this surgical awl is also called "sword needle" which was used to eliminate pus and sputum. This is one of the 78 surgical appliances in traditional Chinese medicine surgery of the late Qing Dynasty which were displayed in this museum and collected by purchasing, solicitation and donation and so on. It is basically well-preserved. There are some signs of use on the edge, with some rust spots slightly covered on the body.
Preserved in Chinese Medical Association/ Museum of Chinese Medicine, Shanghai University of Traditional Chinese Medicine

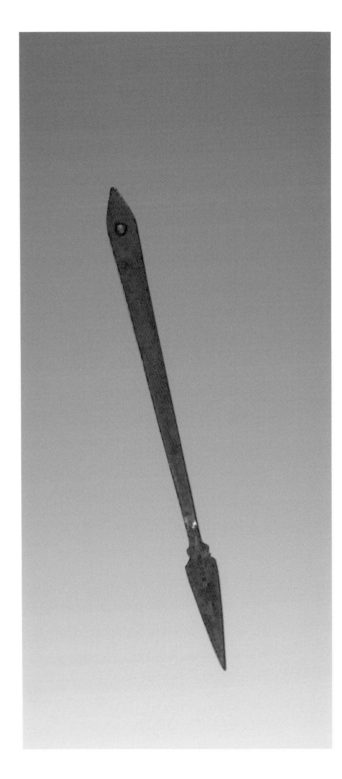

外科簇尖刺锥

清

铁质

通长 11.1 厘米

刃：长 2.5 厘米，宽 0.7 厘米

柄：宽 0.7 厘米

Surgical Awl with Pointed Tip

Qing Dynasty

Iron

Length 11.1 cm

Blade: Length 2.5 cm/ Width 0.7 cm

Hilt: Width 0.7 cm

长锥形，为外科手术用具。此锥为双刃，《喉
科心法》称"剑针"，用做"备通脓管之用，
取其迅速，痰包亦用此破"。这是该馆通过
自购、征集、受捐等方式收藏展出的 78 件
清末中医外科手术用具之一。保存基本完好，
刃部有使用痕迹，刀身可见轻微锈斑。

中华医学会／上海中医药大学医史博物馆藏

This long awl-like knife is a tool for surgical
operations. This awl has two edges. In the
book *Hou Ke Xin Fa* (a medical book on
laryngology), this surgical awl is also called
"sword needle" which was used to eliminate
pus and sputum. This is one of the 78 surgical
appliances in traditional Chinese medicine
surgery of the late Qing Dynasty which were
displayed in this museum and collected by
purchasing, solicitation and donation and so on.
It is basically well-preserved. There are some
signs of use on the edge, with some rust spots
slightly covered on the body.

Preserved in Chinese Medical Association/
Museum of Chinese Medicine, Shanghai
University of Traditional Chinese Medicine

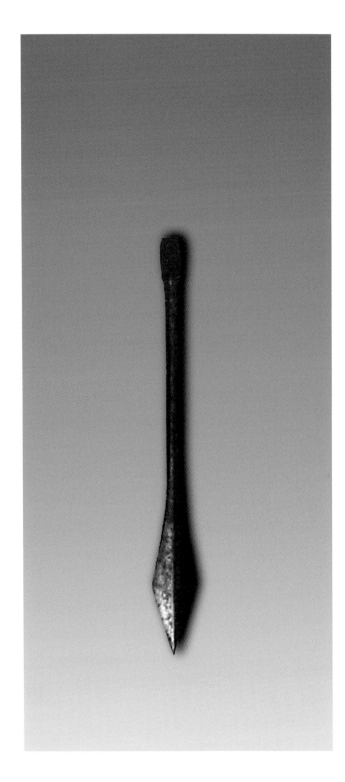

外科簇尖刺锥

清

铁质

通长 9.6 厘米

刃：长 1.7 厘米，宽 1 厘米

柄：宽 0.3 厘米

Surgical Awl with Pointed Tip

Qing Dynasty

Iron

Length 9.6 cm

Blade: Length 1.7 cm/ Width 1 cm

Hilt: Width 0.3 cm

长锥形，为外科手术用具。此锥为双刃，《喉科心法》称"剑针"，用做"备通脓管之用，取其迅速，痰包亦用此破"。这是该馆通过自购、征集、受捐等方式收藏展出的78件清末中医外科手术用具之一。保存基本完好，刃部有使用痕迹，刀身可见有轻微锈斑。

中华医学会／上海中医药大学医史博物馆藏

This long awl-like knife is a tool for surgical operations. This awl has two edges. In the book *Hou Ke Xin Fa* (a medical book on laryngology), this surgical awl is also called "sword needle" which was used to eliminate pus and sputum. This is one of the 78 surgical appliances in traditional Chinese medicine surgery of the late Qing Dynasty which were displayed in this museum and collected by purchasing, solicitation and donation and so on. It is basically well-preserved. There are some signs of use on the edge, with some rust spots slightly covered on the body.

Preserved in Chinese Medical Association/ Museum of Chinese Medicine, Shanghai University of Traditional Chinese Medicine

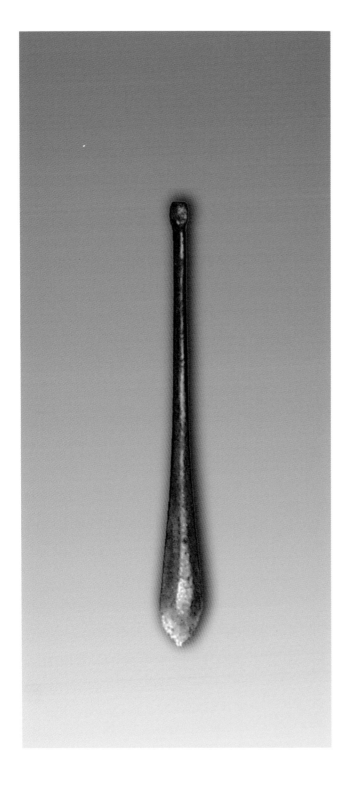

外科簇尖刺锥

清

铁质

通长 8.5 厘米

刃：长 0.8 厘米，宽 0.9 厘米

柄：宽 0.3 厘米

Surgical Awl with Pointed Tip

Qing Dynasty

Iron

Length 8.5 cm

Blade: Length 0.8 cm/ Width 0.9 cm

Hilt: Width 0.3 cm

长锥形，为外科手术用具。此锥为双刃，《喉科心法》称"剑针"，用做"备通脓管之用，取其迅速，痰包亦用此破"。这是该馆通过自购、征集、受捐等方式收藏展出的78件清末中医外科手术用具之一。保存基本完好，刃部有使用痕迹，刀身可见有轻微锈斑。

中华医学会/上海中医药大学医史博物馆藏

This long awl-like knife is a tool for surgical operations. This awl has two edges. In the book *Hou Ke Xin Fa* (a medical book on laryngology), this surgical awl is also called "sword needle" which was used to eliminate pus and sputum. This is one of the 78 surgical appliances in traditional Chinese medicine surgery of the late Qing Dynasty which were displayed in this museum and collected by purchasing, solicitation and donation and so on. It is basically well-preserved. There are some signs of use on the edge, with some rust spots slightly covered on the body.

Preserved in Chinese Medical Association/ Museum of Chinese Medicine, Shanghai University of Traditional Chinese Medicine

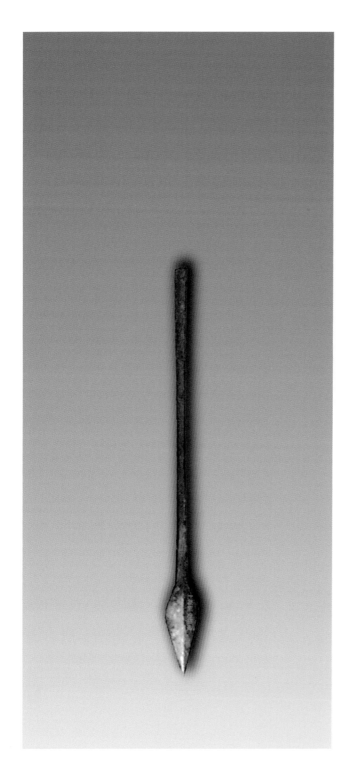

外科簇尖刺锥

清

铁质

通长 8.3 厘米

刃：长 1.3 厘米，宽 0.8 厘米

柄：宽 0.3 厘米

Surgical Awl with Pointed Tip

Qing Dynasty

Iron

Length 8.3 cm

Blade: Length 1.3 cm/ Width 0.8 cm

Hilt: Width 0.3 cm

长锥形，为外科手术用具。此锥为双刃，《喉科心法》称"剑针"，用做"备通脓管之用，取其迅速，痰包亦用此破"。这是该馆通过自购、征集、受捐等方式收藏展出的78件清末中医外科手术用具之一。保存基本完好，刃部有使用痕迹，刀身可见有轻微锈斑。

中华医学会 / 上海中医药大学医史博物馆藏

This long awl-like knife is a tool for surgical operations. This awl has two edges. In the book *Hou Ke Xin Fa* (a medical book on laryngology), this surgical awl is also called "sword needle" which was used to eliminate pus and sputum. This is one of the 78 surgical appliances in traditional Chinese medicine surgery of the late Qing Dynasty which were displayed in this museum and collected by purchasing, solicitation and donation and so on. It is basically well-preserved. There are some signs of use on the edge, with some rust spots slightly covered on the body.

Preserved in Chinese Medical Association/ Museum of Chinese Medicine, Shanghai University of Traditional Chinese Medicine

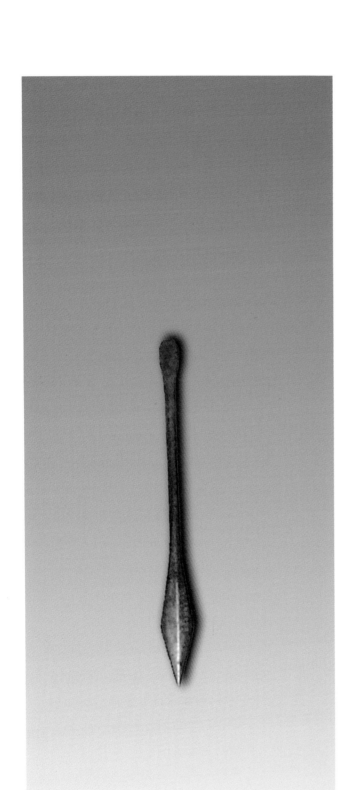

外科簇尖刺锥

清

铁质

通长 7.6 厘米

刃：长 1.4 厘米，宽 0.8 厘米

柄：宽 0.3 厘米

Surgical Awl with Pointed Tip

Qing Dynasty

Iron

Length 7.6 cm

Blade: Length 1.4 cm/ Width 0.8 cm

Hilt: Width 0.3 cm

长锥形，为外科手术用具。此锥为双刃，《喉科心法》称"剑针"，用做"备通脓管之用，取其迅速，痰包亦用此破"。这是该馆通过自购、征集、受捐等方式收藏展出的78件清末中医外科手术用具之一。保存基本完好，刃部有使用痕迹，刀身可见有轻微锈斑。

中华医学会/上海中医药大学医史博物馆藏

This long awl-like knife is a tool for surgical operations. This awl has two edges. In the book *Hou Ke Xin Fa* (a medical book on laryngology), this surgical awl is also called "sword needle" which was used to eliminate pus and sputum. This is one of the 78 surgical appliances in traditional Chinese medicine surgery of the late Qing Dynasty which were displayed in this museum and collected by purchasing, solicitation and donation and so on. It is basically well-preserved. There are some signs of use on the edge, with some rust spots slightly covered on the body.
Preserved in Chinese Medical Association/ Museum of Chinese Medicine, Shanghai University of Traditional Chinese Medicine

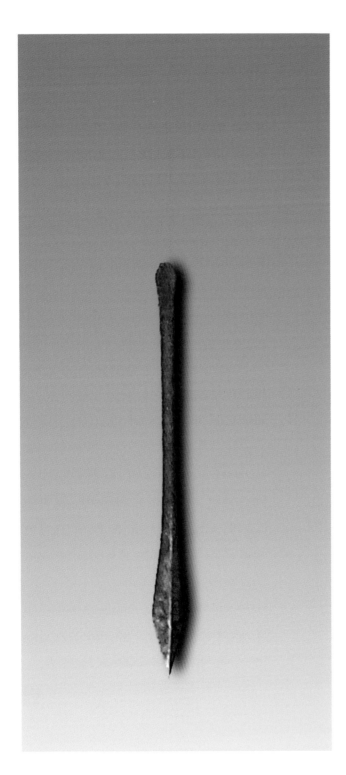

外科簇尖刺锥

清

铁质

通长 6.6 厘米

刃：长 1.1 厘米，宽 0.6 厘米

柄：宽 0.3 厘米

Surgical Awl with Pointed Tip

Qing Dynasty

Iron

Length 6.6 cm

Blade: Length 1.1 cm/ Width 0.6 cm

Hilt: Width 0.3 cm

长锥形，为外科手术用具。此锥为双刃，《喉科心法》称"剑针"，用做"备通脓管之用，取其迅速，痰包亦用此破"。这是该馆通过自购、征集、受捐等方式收藏展出的 78 件清末中医外科手术用具之一。保存基本完好，刃部有使用痕迹，刀身可见有轻微锈斑。

中华医学会 / 上海中医药大学医史博物馆藏

This long awl-like knife is a tool for surgical operations. This awl has two edges. In the book *Hou Ke Xin Fa* (a medical book on laryngology), this surgical awl is also called "sword needle" which was used to eliminate pus and sputum. This is one of the 78 surgical appliances in traditional Chinese medicine surgery of the late Qing Dynasty which were displayed in this museum and collected by purchasing, solicitation and donation and so on. It is basically well-preserved. There are some signs of use on the edge, with some rust spots slightly covered on the body.

Preserved in Chinese Medical Association/ Museum of Chinese Medicine, Shanghai University of Traditional Chinese Medicine

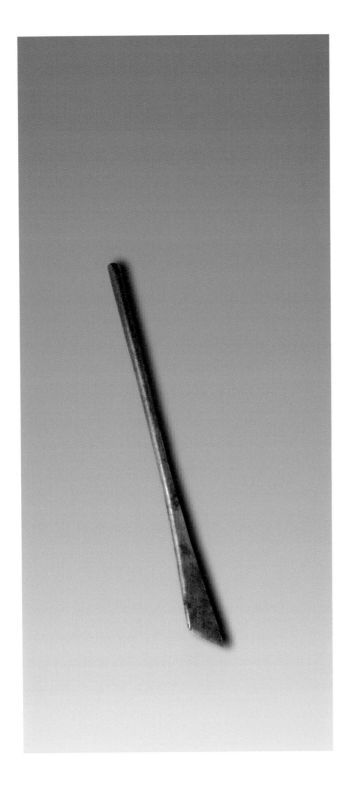

外科斜刃刀

清

铁质

通长 10.3 厘米

柄：径 0.3 厘米

刃：长 1.2 厘米

Surgical Knife with Oblique Edge

Qing Dynasty

Iron

Length 10.3 cm

Hilt: Diameter 0.3 cm

Blade: Length 1.2 cm

直形，为外科手术用具。斜刃刀是中医外科最基本的手术用具，主要用做切开疮痈。这是该馆接受卢大均中医师捐献而收藏的一组清末中医外科手术用具之一。保存基本完好，钩尖处有使用痕迹，手柄处有轻微锈斑。

中华医学会／上海中医药大学医史博物馆藏

The straight scalpel was used as a surgical instrument. Surgical scalpels with oblique blade are the most basic surgical instrument for incising skin ulcer. This is one of a series of traditional Chinese medical surgical instruments in the late Qing Dynasty donated by practitioner Lu Dajun of traditional Chinese medicine. It is preserved in basically good condition. The point of the hook shows sign of use, while slight rust appears on the hilt.

Preserved in Chinese Medical Association/ Museum of Chinese Medicine, Shanghai University of Traditional Chinese Medicine

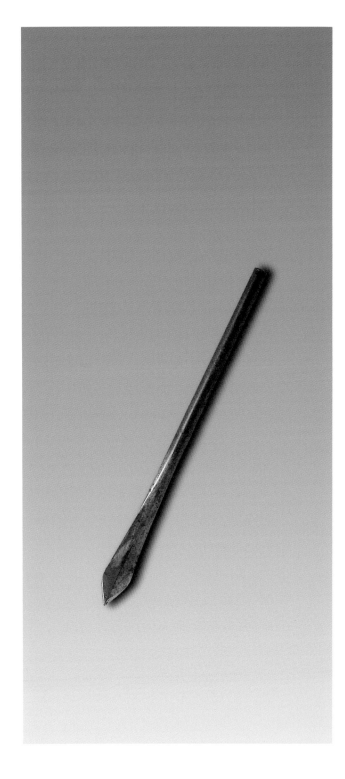

外科簇尖刺锥

清

铁质

通长 11.07 厘米

刃：长 1.34 厘米，宽 1.04 厘米

柄：宽 0.4 厘米

Surgical Awl with Pointed Tip

Qing Dynasty

Iron

Length 11.07 cm

Blade: Length 1.34 cm/ Width 1.04 cm

Hilt: Width 0.4 cm

长锥形，为外科手术用具。此锥为双刃，《喉科心法》称"剑针"，用做"备通脓管之用，取其迅速，痰包亦用此破"。这是该馆接受卢大均中医师捐献而收藏的一组清末中医外科手术用具之一。保存基本完好，刃部有使用痕迹，刀身可见轻微锈斑。

中华医学会 / 上海中医药大学医史博物馆藏

This long awl-like knife is a tool for surgical operations. This awl has two edges. In the book *Hou Ke Xin Fa* (a medical book on laryngology), this surgical awl is also called "sword needle" which was used to eliminate pus and sputum. This is one of a series of traditional Chinese medical surgical instruments in the late Qing Dynasty donated by practitioner Lu Dajun of traditional Chinese medicine. It is basically well-preserved. There are some signs of use on the edge, with some rust spots slightly covered on the body.

Preserved in Chinese Medical Association/ Museum of Chinese Medicine, Shanghai University of Traditional Chinese Medicine

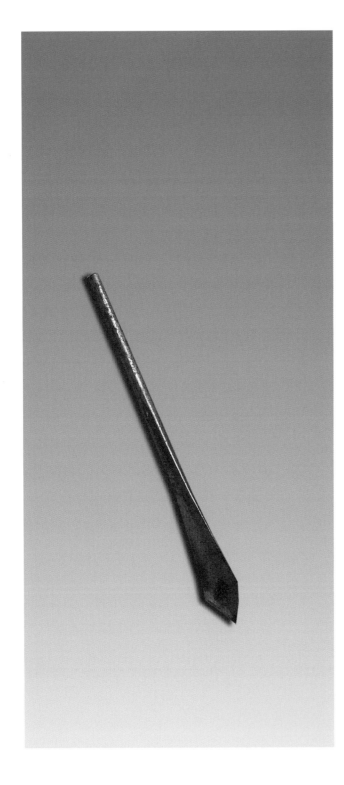

外科簇尖刺锥

清

铁质

通长 11.96 厘米

刃：长 1.3 厘米，宽 1.3 厘米

柄：宽 0.4 厘米

Surgical Awl with Pointed Tip

Qing Dynasty

Iron

Length 11.96 cm

Blade: Length 1.3 cm/ Width 1.3 cm

Hilt: Width 0.4 cm

长锥形，为外科手术用具。此锥为双刃，《喉科心法》称"剑针"，用做"备通脓管之用，取其迅速，痰包亦用此破"。这是该馆接受卢大均中医师捐献而收藏的一组清末中医外科手术用具之一。保存基本完好，刃部有使用痕迹，刀身可见有轻微锈斑。

中华医学会 / 上海中医药大学医史博物馆藏

This long awl-like knife is a tool for surgical operations. This awl has two edges. In the book *Hou Ke Xin Fa* (a medical book on laryngology), this surgical awl is also called "sword needle" which was used to eliminate pus and sputum. This is one of a series of traditional Chinese medical surgical instruments in the late Qing Dynasty donated by practitioner Lu Dajun of traditional Chinese medicine. It is basically well-preserved. There are some signs of use on the edge, with some rust spots slightly covered on the body.

Preserved in Chinese Medical Association/ Museum of Chinese Medicine, Shanghai University of Traditional Chinese Medicine

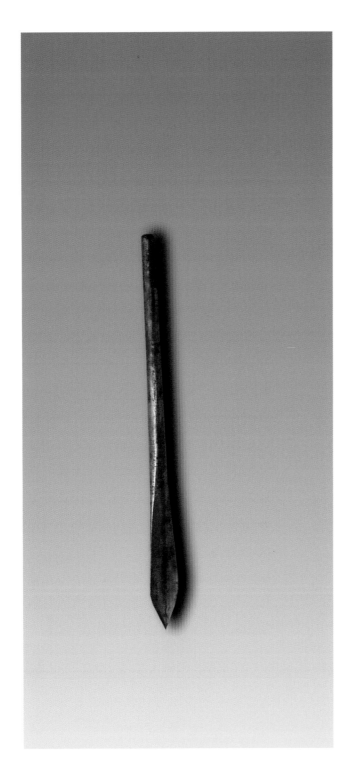

外科簇尖刺锥

清

铁质

通长 10.25 厘米

刃：长 0.96 厘米，宽 0.88 厘米

柄：宽 0.4 厘米

Surgical Awl with Pointed Tip

Qing Dynasty

Iron

Length 10.25 cm

Blade: Length 0.96 cm/ Width 0.88 cm

Hilt: Width 0.4 cm

长锥形，为外科手术用具。此锥为双刃，《喉科心法》称"剑针"，用做"备通脓管之用，取其迅速，痰包亦用此破"。这是该馆接受卢大均中医师捐献而收藏的一组清末中医外科手术用具之一。保存基本完好，刃部有使用痕迹，刀身可见有轻微锈斑。

中华医学会 / 上海中医药大学医史博物馆藏

This long awl-like knife is a tool for surgical operations. This awl has two edges. In the book *Hou Ke Xin Fa* (a medical book on laryngology), this surgical awl is also called "sword needle" which was used to eliminate pus and sputum. This is one of a series of traditional Chinese medical surgical instruments in the late Qing Dynasty donated by practitioner Lu Dajun of traditional Chinese medicine. It is basically well-preserved. There are some signs of use on the edge, with some rust spots slightly covered on the body.
Preserved in Chinese Medical Association/ Museum of Chinese Medicine, Shanghai University of Traditional Chinese Medicine

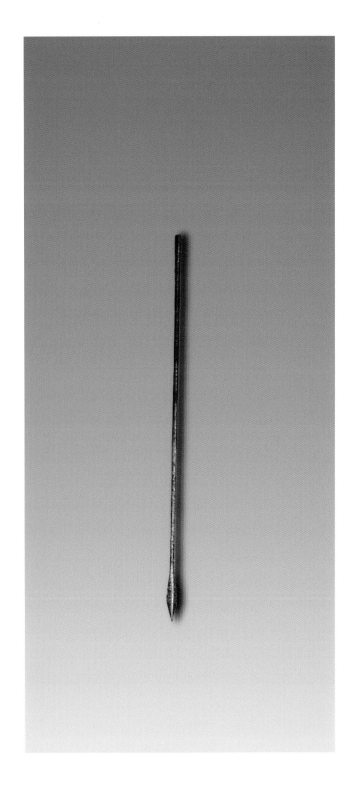

外科尖棱锥

清

铁质

通长 14.3 厘米

棱刃：长 0.8 厘米，宽 0.6 厘米

柄：径 0.3 厘米

Surgical Awl with Sharp and Pyramid-Shaped Tip

Qing Dynasty

Iron

Length 14.3 cm

Blade: Length 0.8 cm/ Width 0.6 cm

Hilt: Diameter 0.3 cm

长锥形，为常用外科手术用具。此锥尖部为四棱形，棱线呈锋刃。《喉科心法》亦称"剑针"，用做"备通脓管之用，取其迅速，痰包亦用此破"。这是该馆通过自购、征集、受捐等方式收藏展出的 78 件清末中医外科手术用具之一。保存基本完好，刃部有使用痕迹，刀身可见轻微锈斑。

中华医学会 / 上海中医药大学医史博物馆藏

This long awl-like knife is a tool for surgical operations. This tip of this awl is like quadrangular pyramid shape, and the ridge shows its sharp edge. In the book *Hou Ke Xin Fa* (a medical book on laryngology), this surgical awl is also called "sword needle" which was used to eliminate pus and sputum. This is one of the 78 surgical appliances in traditional Chinese medicine surgery of the late Qing Dynasty which were displayed in this museum and collected by purchaing, solicitation and donation and so on. It is basically well-preserved. There are some signs of use on the edge, with some rust spots slightly covered on the body.

Preserved in Chinese Medical Association/Museum of Chinese Medicine, Shanghai University of Traditional Chinese Medicine

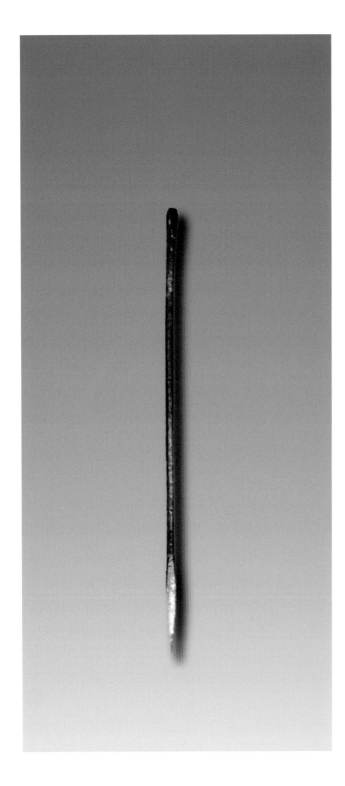

外科尖棱锥

清

铁质

通长 11.9 厘米

棱刃：长 1.7 厘米，宽 0.3 厘米

柄：径 0.3 厘米

Surgical Awl with Sharp and Pyramid-Shaped Tip

Qing Dynasty

Iron

Length 11.9 cm

Blade: Length 1.7 cm/ Width 0.3 cm

Hilt: Diameter 0.3 cm

长锥形，为常用外科手术用具。此锥尖部为三棱形，棱线呈锋刃。《喉科心法》亦称"剑针"，用做"备通脓管之用，取其迅速，痰包亦用此破"。这是该馆通过自购、征集、受捐等方式收藏展出的78件清末中医外科手术用具之一。保存基本完好，刃部有使用痕迹，刀身可见有轻微锈斑。

中华医学会/上海中医药大学医史博物馆藏

This long awl-like knife is a tool for surgical operations. This tip of this awl is like quadrangular pyramid shape, and the ridge shows its sharp edge. In the book *Hou Ke Xin Fa* (a medical book on laryngology), this surgical awl is also called "sword needle" which was used to eliminate pus and sputum. This is one of the 78 surgical appliances in traditional Chinese medicine surgery of the late Qing Dynasty which were displayed in this museum and collected by purchaing, solicitation and donation and so on. It is basically well-preserved. There are some signs of use on the edge, with some rust spots slightly covered on the body. Preserved in Chinese Medical Association/Museum of Chinese Medicine, Shanghai University of Traditional Chinese Medicine

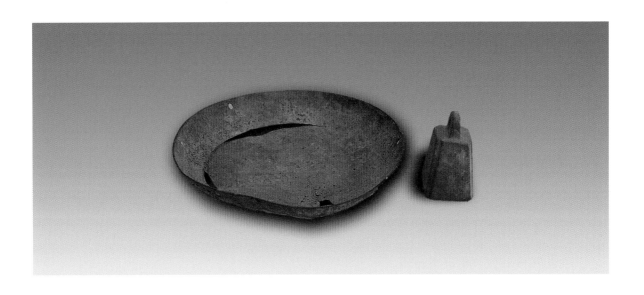

秤

清

铁质

盘：直径 15 厘米

秤锤：通高 5 厘米，重 450 克

一秤盘一秤杆。衡器。有残。陕西省长安县征集。

陕西医史博物馆藏

Scale

Qing Dynasty

Iron

Tray: Diameter 15 cm

Counterpoise: Height 5 cm/ Weight 450 g

These are a load tray and a scale beam. It is a weighing apparatus with the tray partially damaged. It was collected from Chang'an County, Shaanxi Province.

Preserved in Shaanxi Museum of Medical History

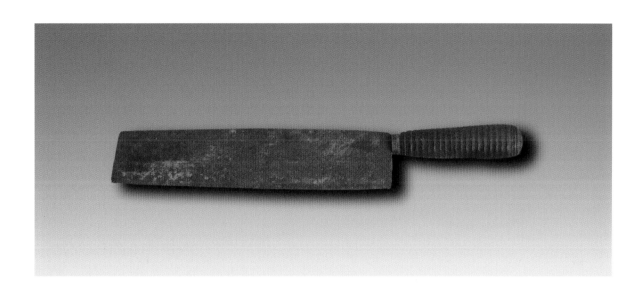

铁刀

清

铁质

长 22.5 厘米，宽 3.5 厘米，重 100 克

长条形刀，较薄，弦纹胶木把。生活用刀具。完整无损。

陕西医史博物馆藏

Iron Knife

Qing Dynasty

Iron

Length 22.5 cm/ Width 3.5 cm/ Weight 100 g

The knife is rectangular and thin, with a string patterned bakelite handle. It is a life appliance which is well-preserved.

Preserved in Shaanxi Museum of Medical History

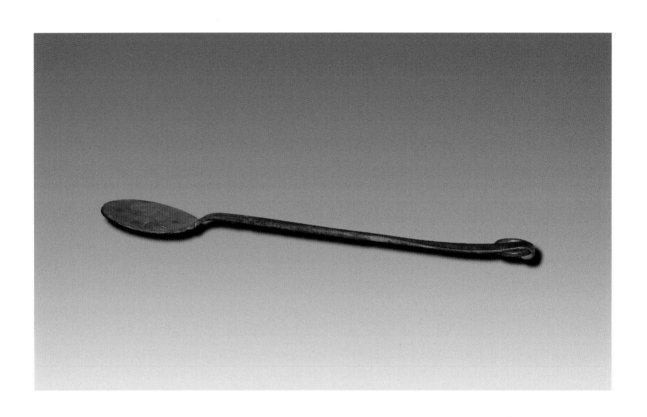

铜铲

清

铜质

长 27 厘米，宽 5 厘米，重 50 克

Copper Shovel

Qing Dynasty

Copper

Length 27 cm/ Width 5 cm/ Weight 50 g

铲头呈圆形，柄为长条形，柄把有一圆环。
生活用具。完整无损。

陕西医史博物馆藏

The scoop is round in the head and the handle is elongated with a circular ring at the end. It is a life appliance which is well-preserved.

Preserved in Shaanxi Museum of Medical History

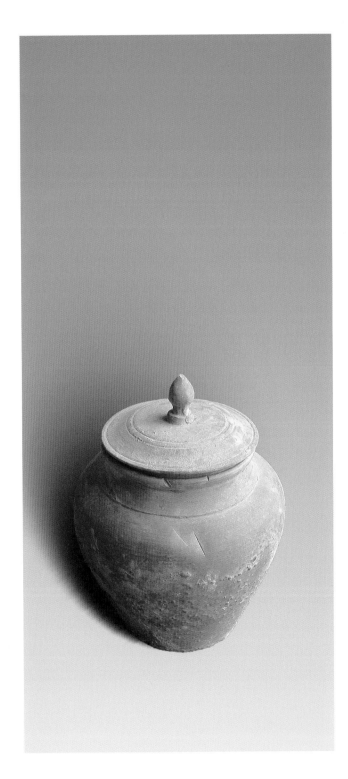

锡罐

民国时期

锡质

口径 6.5 厘米，腹径 9.7 厘米，高 9.7 厘米

Tin Can

Republican Period

Tin

Mouth Diameter 6.5 cm/ Belly Diameter 9.7 cm/

Height 9.7 cm

敞口，束颈，斜肩，肩刻弦纹一周，鼓腹，平底，宝塔钮盖上刻弦纹。盛药工具。

江苏省中医药博物馆藏

The can has a snap-lid, a swelling belly, a straight spout, an arc bridge-shaped handle, a flat bottom and a pogada-shaped button. It was used for decocting Chinese medicine.

Preserved in Jiangsu Museum of Traditional Chinese Medicine

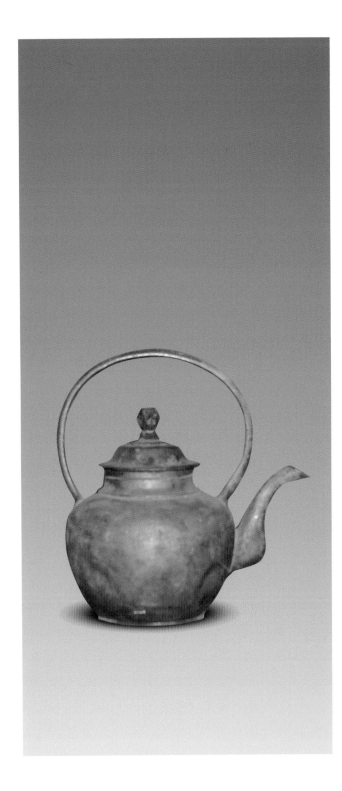

铜壶

清

铜质

口径 4.9 厘米，底径 6 厘米，通高 14 厘米，重 500 克

Copper Pot

Qing Dynasty

Copper

Mouth Diameter 4.9 cm/ Bottom Diameter 6 cm/ Height 14 cm/ Weight 500 g

子母口，圆腹，平底，带一盖，上腹有一水流，
一壶把。生活用器。完整无损。

陕西医史博物馆藏

The pot has a snap-lid, a round belly and a
flat bottom. There are a spout and a handle on
the upper belly. It is a life appliance which is
well-preserved.

Preserved in Shaanxi Museum of Medical History

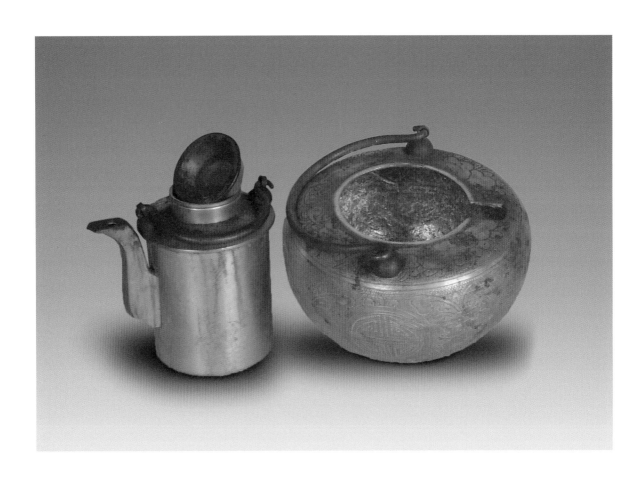

铝参壶

清

铝质

壶径 9.2 厘米，通高 6.85 厘米

Aluminum Pot for Cooking Ginseng Soup

Qing Dynasty

Aluminum

Pot Diameter 9.2 cm/ Height 6.85 cm

壶状，用于蒸人参汤。该藏工艺精细，由内、外壶套置而成，内外壶均有铜制提梁，表面刻有福禄寿图案，底部有"潮阳颜义和正老店点铜"款识。1955年入藏。保存完好。

中华医学会／上海中医药大学医史博物馆藏

The utensil is in the shape of a pot, utilized for cooking ginsen soup. Designed with sophisticated craft, it is composed of an inner pot and an outer pot, both of which have copper handles. Patterns about prosperity, promotion and longevity are on its surface. There is inscription reading "Chao Yang Yan Yi He Zheng Lao Dian Dian Tong" on the bottom showing its origin. It was collected in 1955 and is preserved well.

Preserved in Chinese Medical Association/ Museum of Chinese Medicine, Shanghai University of Traditional Chinese Medicine

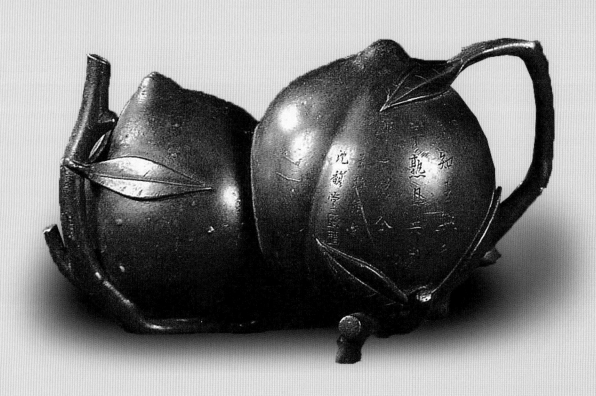

双桃锡酒壶

清

锡质

长 18 厘米，高 12 厘米

双桃并蒂状。款为"沈廷桂制"。设计精巧而科学，可用于温酒。

上海中医药博物馆藏

Tin Flagon in the Shape of Two Peaches

Qing Dynasty

Tin

Length 18 cm/ Height 12 cm

The tin flagon looks like a double peach side by side. The inscription reading "Shen Ting Gui Zhi" (meaning "made by Shen Tinggui"). It is designed with sophisticated and scientific craft. It can be used to heat wine.

Preserved in Chinese Medical Association/Museum of Chinese Medicine, Shanghai University of Traditional Chinese Medicine

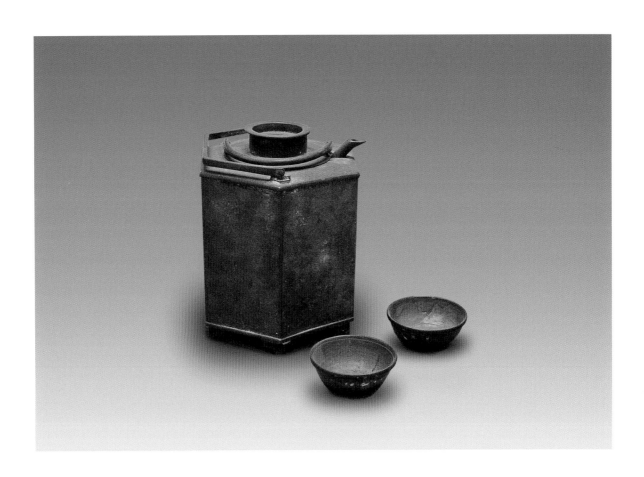

温酒器

清

铜质

高 7 厘米

Utensil for Heating Wine

Qing Dynasty

Copper

Height 7 cm

六角形，器身呈柱状，四足，中间的壶内盛酒，在内、外层之间的间隙盛装热水，用于温热壶中的冷酒，可使人不致伤胃。由民间征集。

成都中医药大学中医药传统文化博物馆藏

The body is a hexagonal column with four feet. The inner utensil is a wine pot and the interlayer can be filled with hot water. It is used to heat the cool wine to protect the stomach. It was collected from the folk.

Preserved in Museum of Traditional Chinese Medicine Culture, Chengdu University of Traditional Chinese Medicine

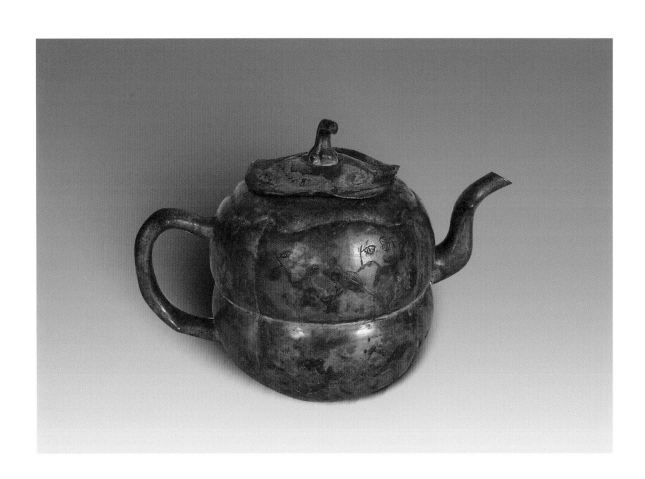

铝茶壶

清

铝质

宽 19.8 厘米，通高 13.5 厘米

Aluminum Tea Pot

Qing Dynasty

Aluminum

Width 19.8 cm/ Height 13.5 cm

茶壶状，为茶具。该藏造型自然纯朴，壶身
形如南瓜，表面浅刻有花鸟图案。底部有款
识"沈存周"等。1957 年入藏。保存基本完好。

中华医学会 / 上海中医药大学医史博物馆藏

The pot is a tea set. It is made with natural and
simple craft and designed with paintings of flowers
and birds. The utensil resembles a pumpkin. There
are characters reading "Shen Cunzhou" inscribed
on the bottom. It was collected in 1957 and is
basically well-preserved.

Preserved in Chinese Medical Association/
Museum of Chinese Medicine, Shanghai
University of Traditional Chinese Medicine

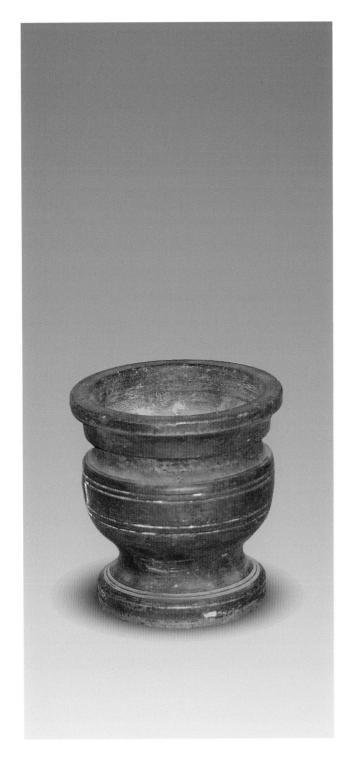

铜杯

清

铜质

重 500 克

平口沿，鼓腹，倒喇叭座，腹有弦纹。食器。
完整无损。

陕西医史博物馆藏

Copper Cup

Qing Dynasty

Copper

Weight 500 g

The mouth edge is flat. The belly is swelling.
The pedestal resembles an inverted horn. There
is string pattern on the belly. It is a well-
preserved food container.

Preserved in Shaanxi Museum of Medical History

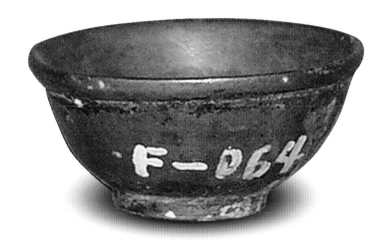

铜酒杯

清

铜质

口径 4.5 厘米，底径 2 厘米，通高 2.2 厘米，重 50 克

酒盅状，斜腹，圈足。酒器。完整无损。陕西省咸阳市征集。

陕西医史博物馆藏

Copper Wine Cup

Qing Dynasty

Copper

Mouth Diameter 4.5 cm/ Bottom Diameter 2 cm/ Height 2.2 cm/ Weight 50 g

It is a small handleless wine cup, with an oblique belly and a ring foot. It is preserved well. It was collected

from Xianyang City, Shaanxi Province.

Preserved in Shaanxi Museum of Medical History

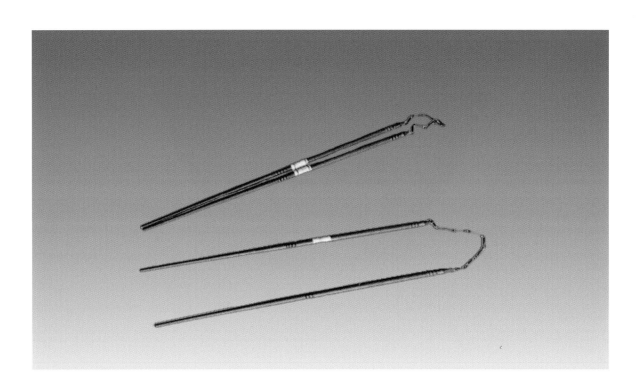

铜箸

清

铜质

长 19.8 厘米，直径 0.1~0.2 厘米

Copper Chopsticks

Qing Dynasty

Copper

Length 19.8 cm/ Diameter 0.1–0.2 cm

两双。该藏两双铜箸形制和规格一致，均为长条形锥体，但箸端圆钝而不尖锐，腰部有几周凸棱为饰，使简单的造型不至于单调，顶端也有凸棱，并以链条将两支箸联成一双，现在仍有这种做法。铜料的质量和色泽使之显得古色古香。

中国箸文化陈列馆藏

The two pairs are of the same shape and specification. Both of them are rectangular and subuliform. The ends of the chopsticks are designed round and blunt. There are several ridges decorating the wrists, simple but not boring. There are also several ridges on the top part, on which there is a chain linking every two chopsticks together. This craft is still practiced today. The quality and the color of the copper make it of antique beauty.

Preserved in China Chopsticks Culture Museum

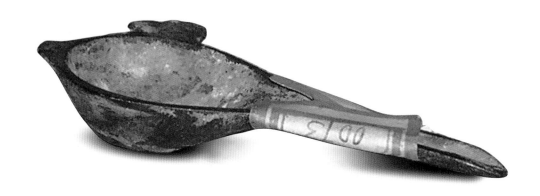

小铜勺

清

铜质

长 7.5 厘米，宽 3.5 厘米，重 1 克

鸟状勺形。生活器具。完整无损。

陕西医史博物馆藏

Small Copper Spoon

Qing Dynasty

Copper

Length 7.5 cm/ Width 3.5 cm/ Weight 1 g

The spoon is designed in the shape of a bird. It is a well-preserved life appliance.

Preserved in Shaanxi Museum of Medical History

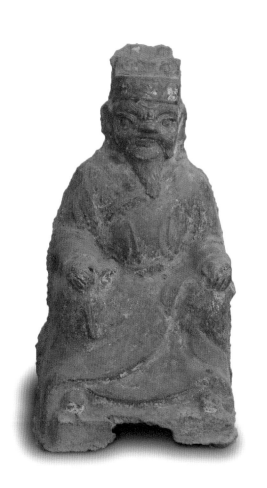

铁像

清

铁质

底长 19 厘米，宽 16 厘米，通高 40 厘米，
重 8000 克

全身坐像，双手抱膝，头带官帽。宗教造像。
完整无损。

陕西医史博物馆藏

Iron Statue

Qing Dynasty

Iron

Bottom Diameter 19 cm/ Width 16 cm/ Height
40 cm/ Weight 8,000 g

This statue is a sitting man, with two hands
placed on knees and an official hat placed on
the head. It is a well-preserved religious statue.

Preserved in Shaanxi Museum of Medical History

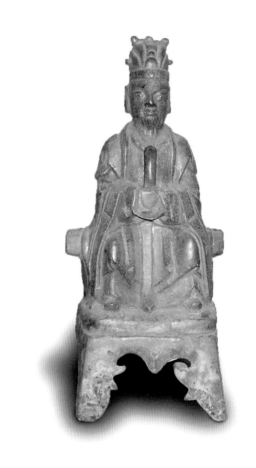

铜像

清

铜质

通高 27.5 厘米，重 1150 克

全身坐像，头戴帽，四齿方形底座，背有"王大口平八"字样。宗教佛像。完整无损。

陕西医史博物馆藏

Copper Statue

Qing Dynasty

Copper

Height 27.5 cm/ Weight 1,150 g

The statue is in a sitting position, with a hat on the head and a square pedestal with four tooth-like feet. There are characters inscribed on its back. It is a well preserved religious statue.

Preserved in Shaanxi Museum of Medical History

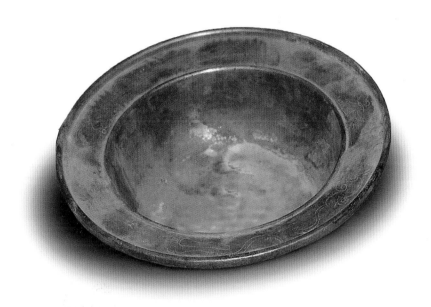

铜盆

清

铜质

口径 11.5 厘米，底径 5.5 厘米，通高 3.2 厘米，平口沿宽 2 厘米，重 150 克

口沿内卷，斜腹，平底。食器。完整无损。陕西省咸阳市征集。

陕西医史博物馆藏

Copper Basin

Qing Dynasty

Copper

Mouth Diameter 11.5 cm/ Bottom Diameter 5.5 cm/ Height 3.2 cm/ Width of the Flat Mouth Edge 2 cm/ Weight 150 g

The mouth edge is curly inward. There is an oblique belly and a flat bottom. It is a dinning appliance which is well-preserved. It was collected from Xianyang City, Shaanxi Province.

Preserved in Shaanxi Museum of Medical History

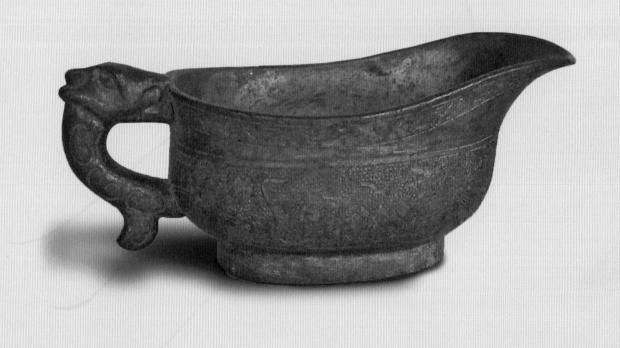

铜刻花匜

清

铜质

长 5.5 厘米，宽 1.02 厘米，通高 4 厘米

匜状，用于盛水。该藏表面浅雕有古琴、瓜、叶等图案，雕工精细，造型美观。1959 年入藏。保存基本完好。

中华医学会 / 上海中医药大学医史博物馆藏

Copper Gourd-shaped Ladle with Engraved Designs

Qing Dynasty

Copper

Length 5.5 cm/ Width 1.02 cm/ Height 4 cm

It is a water container in the shape of a ladle. There are patterns designed in the shape of a seven-stringed plucked instrument, melons and leaves, with fine craft and attractive appearance. It was collected in 1959, and it is basically well-preserved.

Preserved in Chinese Medical Association/Museum of Chinese Medicine, Shanghai University of Traditional Chinese Medicine

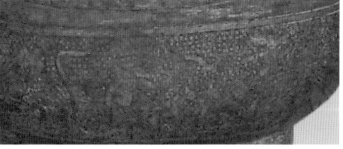

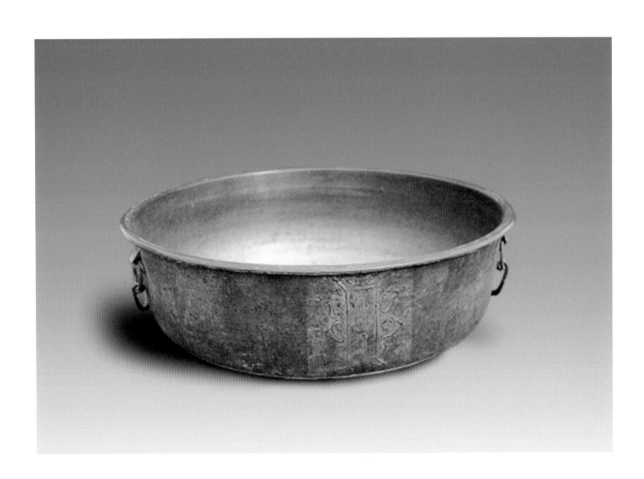

铜盆

清

铜质

口径 77 厘米，底径 58 厘米，高 24 厘米，口沿宽 3 厘米，重 25850 克

Copper Basin

Qing Dynasty

Copper

Mouth Diameter 77 cm/ Bottom Diameter 58 cm/ Height 24 cm/ Width of the Mouth Edge 3 cm/ Weight 25,850 g

敞口，圈足，两侧有环。外壁有"康熙四十年
丑吉日"与"王公子"铭文及花饰。

陕西医史博物馆藏

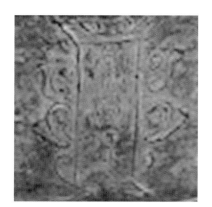

The basin has an open mouth, a ring foot, and ring designs on two sides. There are flower decorations and inscriptions reading "Kang Xi Si Shi Nian Chou Ji Ri" and "Wang Gong Zi" showing a date in the year 1701 and a name title as "Prince Wang".

Preserved in Shaanxi Museum of Medical History

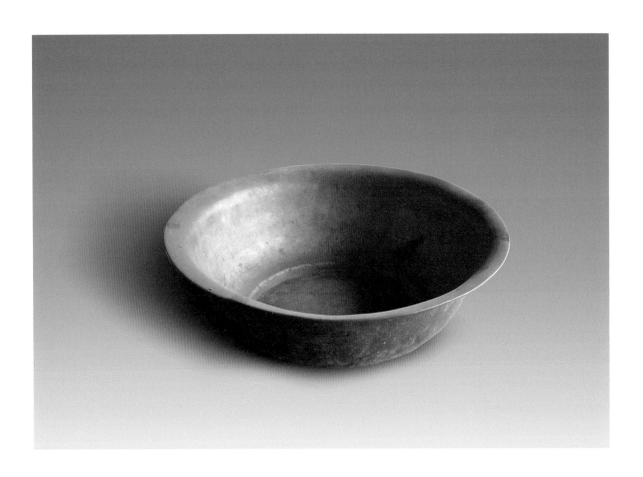

盆

清

铜质

口径 29 厘米，高 9 厘米

Basin

Qing Dynasty

Copper

Mouth Diameter 29 cm/ Height 9 cm

敞口，平底，腹微敛。器物由黄铜制成，腹部有一补丁痕迹，为日常的清洁卫生用具。由民间征集。

　　成都中医药大学中医药传统文化博物馆藏

The basin has an open mouth, and a flat bottom, a slightly oblique belly. It is made from brass. There is a patch on the belly. It is an appliance utilized for daily cleaning and health care. It was collected from the folk.

Preserved in Museum of Traditional Chinese Medicine Culture, Chengdu University of Traditional Chinese Medicine

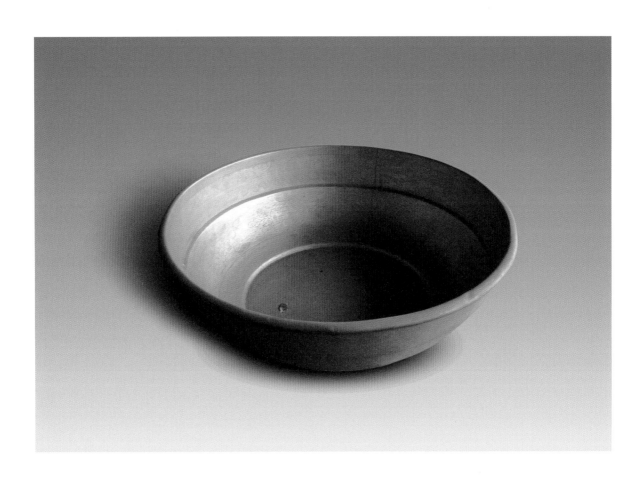

盆

清

铜质

口径 35 厘米，高 10 厘米

Basin

Qing Dynasty

Copper

Mouth Diameter 35 cm/ Height 10 cm

卷口，直肩，平底，腹微敛。盆内錾刻卷云
纹和花卉纹饰，器物造型匀称，色泽光润，
保存完好。盆为洗面用具，在人们日常卫生
保健方面具有广泛用途。由上海市文物商店
征集。

　　成都中医药大学中医药传统文化博物馆藏

The rim of the mouth is curly. It has an upright
shoulder, a flat bottom, and a slightly oblique
belly. There are curly cloud patterns and flower
patterns designed on the inner wall. The basin
is designed in good proportion with bright
luster. It is a washing utensil preserved well and
widely used for health care. It was collected
from an antique shop in Shanghai City.

Preserved in Museum of Traditional Chinese
Medicine Culture, Chengdu University of Traditional
Chinese Medicine

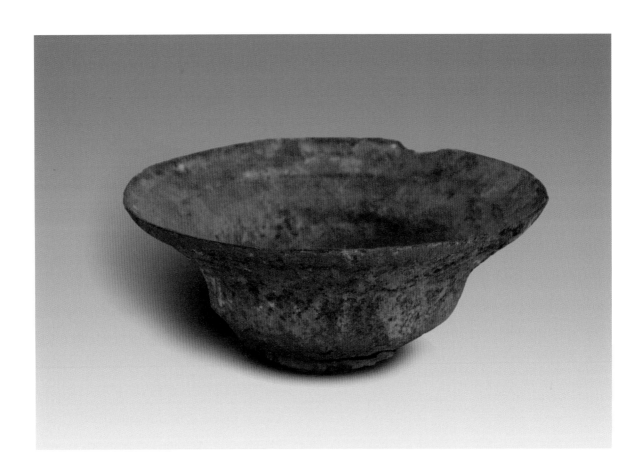

铁盆

清

铁质

口径 21.8 厘米，底径 7.7 厘米，通高 8.7 厘米，重 1300 克

Iron Basin

Qing Dynasty

Iron

Mouth Diameter 21.8 cm/ Bottom Diameter 7.7 cm/ Height 8.7 cm/ Weight 1,300 g

敞口，斜肩，圈足。盛贮器。完整无损。陕西省澄城县善化乡征集。

陕西医史博物馆藏

The basin has an open mouth, an oblique shoulder, and a ring foot. It is a well-preserved storage container. It was collected from Shanhua Village, Chengcheng County, Shaanxi Province.

Preserved in Shaanxi Museum of Medical History

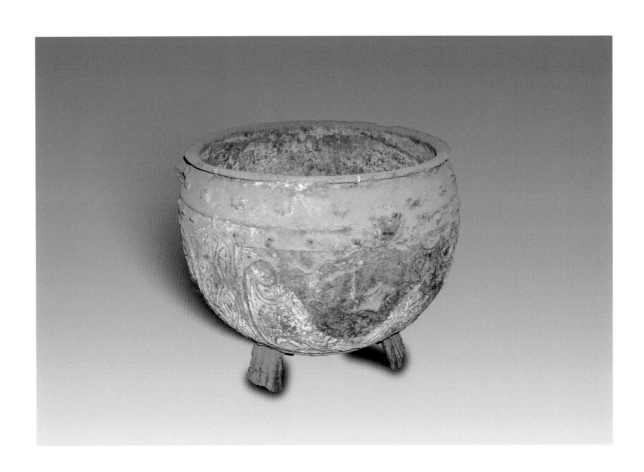

圆铁盒

清

铁质

直径 67 厘米，通高 64 厘米，足高 12 厘米

Round Iron Container

Qing Dynasty

Iron

Diameter 67 cm/ Height 64 cm/ Height of the Leg 12 cm

圆唇，鼓腹，三扁足，上腹有三耳，一圈花瓣，一圈乳丁，中腹浮雕。此为陕西渭北高原特有的一种煮水器具，民间俗称"铁盒"。盛贮器，口沿稍残。陕西省长安区引镇征集。

陕西医史博物馆藏

This utensil has a round lip, a swelling belly and three flat legs. There are three ears. Patterns of flower petals and tiny nails relief are around the belly. As a unique container for boiling water in northern Shaanxi plateau, it is commonly called "Tie He". It was utilized as a storage container. Part of the mouth edge is damaged. It was collected from Yin Township, Chang'an County, Shaanxi Province.

Preserved in Shaanxi Museum of Medical History

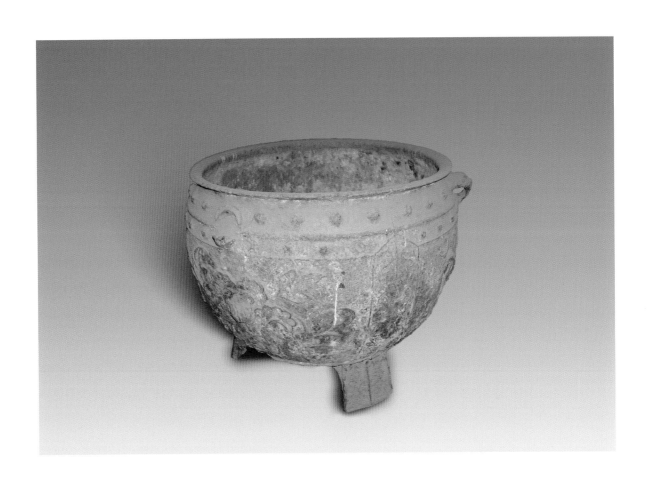

圆铁盒

清

铁质

口径 68 厘米，通高 60 厘米，足高 14 厘米

Round Iron Container

Qing Dynasty

Iron

Mouth Diameter 68 cm/ Height 60 cm/ Height of the Leg 14 cm

圆唇，鼓腹，三扁足，上腹有三耳，一圈花瓣，一圈乳丁浮雕图。此为陕西渭北高原特有的一种煮水器具，民间俗称"铁盒"。盛贮器。口沿稍残。陕西省长安区引镇征集。

陕西医史博物馆藏

This utensil has a round lip, a swelling belly and three flat legs. There are three ears. Patterns of flower petals and tiny nail reliefs are around the belly. As a unique container for boiling water in northern Shaanxi plateau, it is commonly called "Tie He". It was utilized as a storage container. Part of the mouth edge is damaged. It was collected from Yin Township, Chang'an County, Shaanxi Province.

Preserved in Shaanxi Museum of Medical History

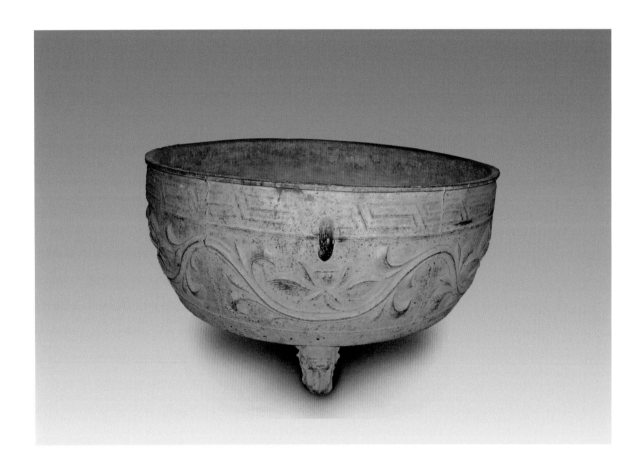

铁盒

清

铁质

长 101 厘米，宽 57 厘米，通高 42.5 厘米

Iron Container

Qing Dynasty

Iron

Length 101 cm/ Width 57 cm/ Weight 42.5 cm

长方形口，直腹，腹上有浮雕，四环耳，四兽足。此为陕西渭北高原特有的一种煮水器具，民间俗称"铁盒"。生活器具。底残少三环。陕西省三原县征集。

陕西医史博物馆藏

This utensil has a rectangular mouth, an upright belly with reliefs on it, four ring-like ears and four beast-shaped feet. As a unique container for boiling water in northern Shaanxi plateau, it is commonly called "Tie He". It is a life appliance. The bottom is damaged, and three rings are missing. It was collected from Sanyuan County, Shaanxi Province.

Preserved in Shaanxi Museum of Medical History

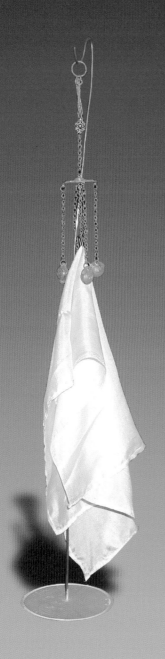

银帕架

清

银质

长 20 厘米，重 30 克

环形链，中间有一圆盘，带四个小铃，中间
小钩。生活卫生器具。完整无损。

陕西医史博物馆藏

Silver Handkerchief Holder

Qing Dynasty

Silver

Length 20 cm/ Weight 30 g

The chains are connected by a ring. There is
a round plate and a hooklet in the middle and
four tiny bells. It is a well-preserved sanitary
apparatus.

Preserved in Shaanxi Museum of Medical History

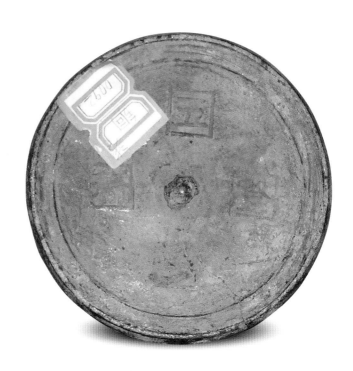

铜镜

清

铜质

直径 10.2 厘米，重 250 克

圆形，镜中心有一圆钮，有铭文"五子登科"。生活器具。有一裂印。

陕西医史博物馆藏

Copper Mirror

Qing Dynasty

Copper

Diameter 10.2 cm/ Weight 250 g

It is a round mirror with a round button in the center and with the Chinese characters reading "Wu Zi Deng Ke" (meaning that five children will manage to pass an imperial examination). It is a life appliance. A crack can be seen on it.

Preserved in Shaanxi Museum of Medical History

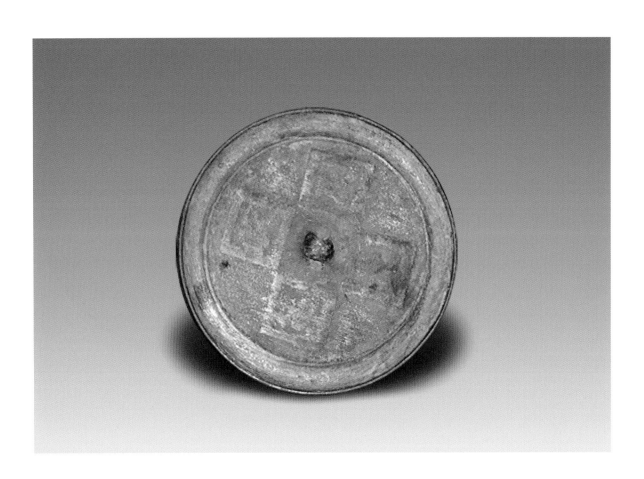

铜镜

清

铜质

直径 10.2 厘米，重 150 克

Copper Mirror

Qing Dynasty

Copper

Diameter 10.2 cm/ Weight 150 g

圆形，镜中心有一圆形钮，外区有一细凸棱，有铭文。生活器具。完整无损。

陕西医史博物馆藏

It is a round mirror with a round button in the center and a fine convex ridge near the rim. There are inscriptions on the back. It is a well-preserved life appliance.

Preserved in Shaanxi Museum of Medical History

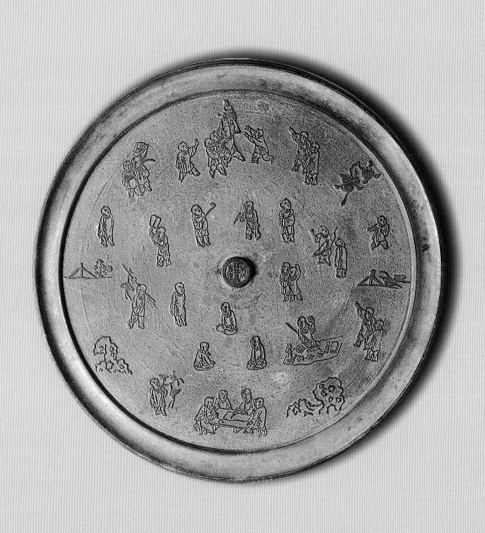

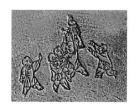

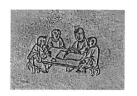

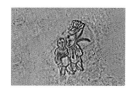

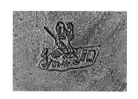

百子图镜

清

铜质

直径 36.5 厘米

圆钮，无钮座。钮上铸"湖州薛晋侯自造"七字，镜背饰三十二个形态不同的天真稚童，其中有五子夺盔，意为"五子夺魁"，有三重三元、莲生贵子、榴开百子等，寓意广泛，皆体现于童子身上所饰之物。此镜形体厚重，制作精细。

中国国家博物馆藏

Mirror with Children Patterns

Qing Dynasty

Copper

Diameter 36.5 cm

There is a round button with no pedestal. There are seven characters "Hu Zhou Xue Jin Hou Zi Zao" inscribed on the button, recording that it was made by Xue Jinhou in Huzhou City, (Zhejiang Province). There are 32 children patterns in different designs decorating the back of the mirror, including five children competing for a helmet (which is a homophone of the first prize), a child holding lotus and sheng (a reed pipe wind instrument), several children circling around the pomegranate, etc. Each pattern embodies a good wish about the offsprings. The mirror weighs heavily and it is made with fine craft.
Preserved in Preserved in National Museum of China

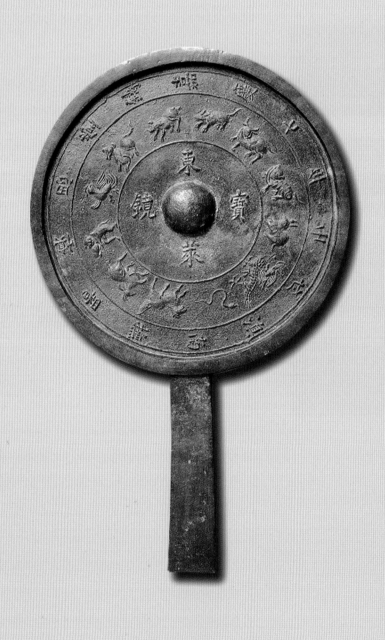

嘉庆慎思堂十二生肖柄镜

清

铜质

直径 17.8 厘米，通柄长 28.1 厘米

圆形带柄，圆钮，无钮座。镜背素地，三周凸弦纹把镜背纹饰分成三区，内区铸铭"东莱宝镜"四字，中区饰十二生肖纹带，外区为"嘉庆七年壬戌滇南抚置慎思堂铸"十四字铭文。嘉庆七年，为公元 1802 年。

中国国家博物馆藏

Mirror of Severance Hall Made in Jiaqing Periods, with Chinese Zodiac Patterns

Qing Dynasty

Copper

Diameter 17.8 cm/ Length of the Handle 28.1 cm

The round mirror has a handle and a round button with no pedestal. The back of the mirror is divided into three regions by three circles of convex string pattern. There are four characters "Dong Lai Bao Jing" and fourteen characters "Jia Qing Qi Nian Ren Xu Dian Nan Fu Zhi Shen Si Tang Zhu" inscribed respectively in the inner and outer regions. The four characters record that it is a precious mirror produced in Donglai (today's Longkou, Shandong). The fourteen characters record that it belongs to Severance Hall in south Yunnan, made in 1802, during Emperor Jiaqing's reign. There are Chinese zodiac patterns inscribed in the middle region.

Preserved in Chinese History Museum

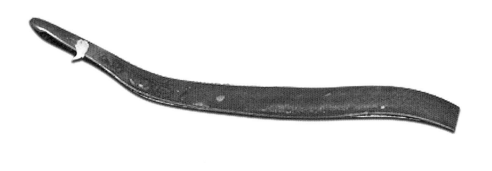

铜发钗

清

铜质

长 9.2 厘米，宽 1 厘米，重 1 克

扁形，弯状呈 S 形。发夹。有残。内蒙古自治区成陵征集。

陕西医史博物馆藏

Copper Hairpin

Qing Dynasty

Copper

Length 9.2 cm/ Width 1 cm/ Weight 1 g

The hairpin is flat and curved in the shape of S. Part of this hairpin is damaged. It was collected from the Mausoleum of Genghis Khan, Inner Mongolia Autonomous Region.

Preserved in Shaanxi Museum of Medical History

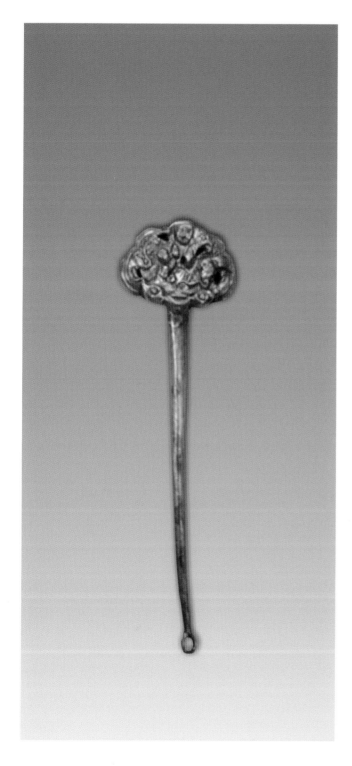

清宫御用鎏金耳挖勺

清

银质鎏金

长 7.1 厘米

清洁耳道用具，器形典雅，做工考究，为清宫或贵族用品。

张雅宗藏

Imperial Gilding Ear Pick

Qing Dynasty

Gilding Silver

Length 7.1 cm

This imperial appliance for picking ears is of elegant shape and exquisite workmanship.

Collected by Zhang Yazong

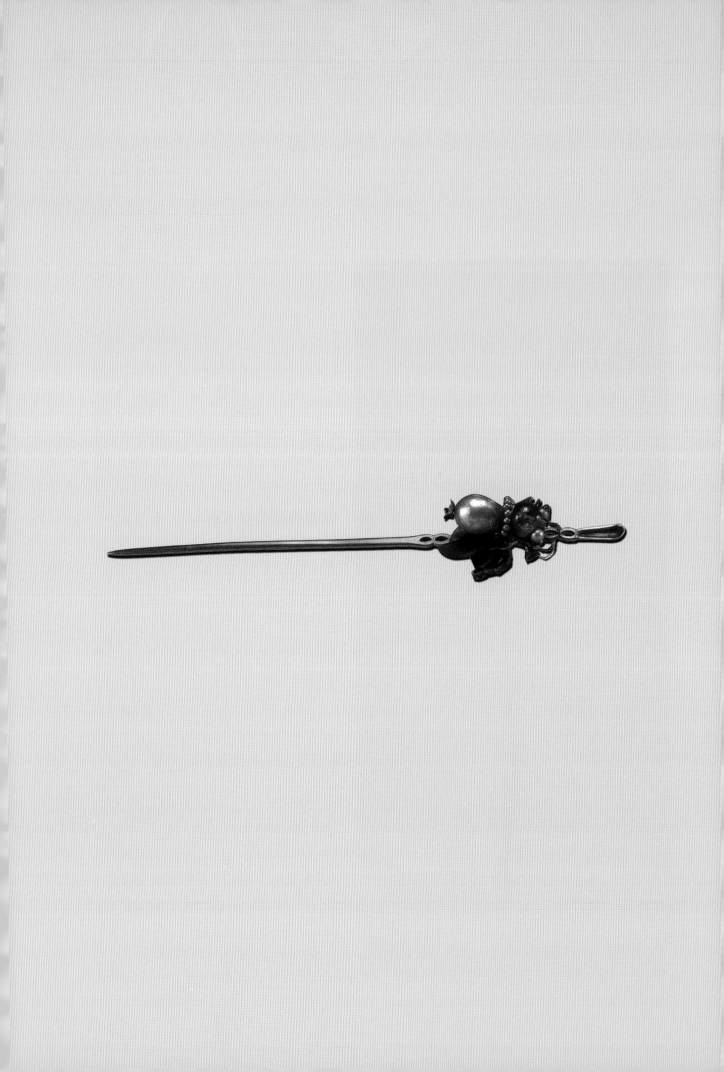

金嵌珠翠耳挖勺簪

清

长 13.5 厘米

清宫后妃首饰，上嵌珍珠一颗。

故宫博物院藏

Gold Ear-picker Hairpin Inlaid with Pearl and Jadeite

Qing Dynasty

Length 13.5 cm

The hairpin is a headgear for concubines in Qing Dynasty Imperial Palace. The hairpin is inlaid with a pearl.

Preserved in The Palace Museum

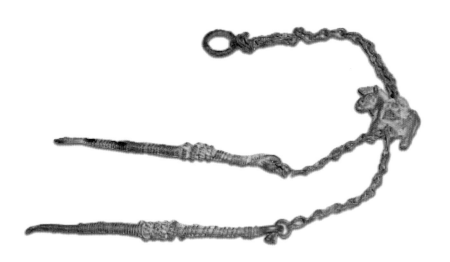

铜二须

清

铜质

长 28.5 厘米，重 18.5 克

二须上有飞马，底端坠有掏耳勺、小镊子各一件。卫生器具。完整无损。

陕西医史博物馆藏

Copper Whisker-like Tools of Two Pieces

Qing Dynasty

Copper

Length 28.5 cm/ Weight 18.5 g

The two whisker-like tools are connected by a horse-shaped decoration. On the other end of each china, there is respectively an earpick and a tweezer. It is a well-preserved sanitary apparatus.

Preserved in Shaanxi Museum of Medical History

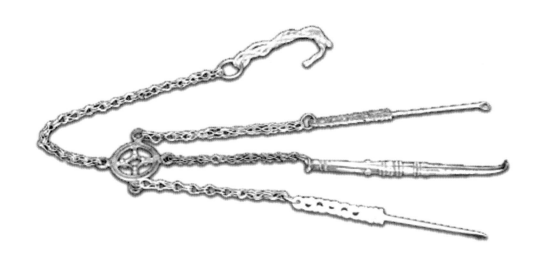

银三须

清

银质

长 30 厘米，重 30 克

环形链，一头有环，带一小镊子、掏耳勺、剔牙棒。卫生器具。完整无损。

陕西医史博物馆藏

Silver Whisker-like Tools of Three Pieces

Qing Dynasty

Silver

Length 30 cm/ Weight 30 g

The three tools are connected by a ring at one end. On the other end of each chain, there are respectively a pair of tweezers, an earpick, and a toothpick. It is a well-preserved sanitary apparatus.

Preserved in Shaanxi Museum of Medical History

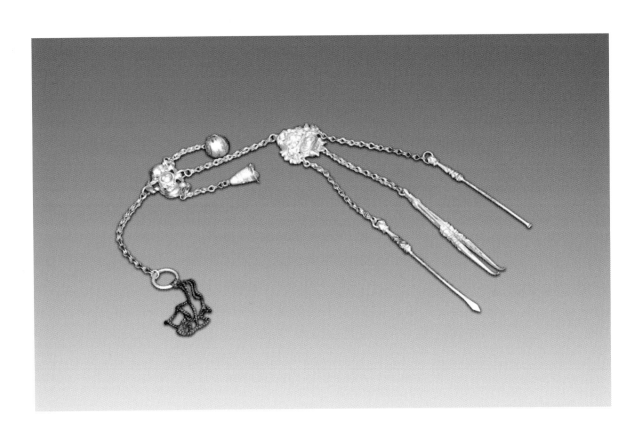

银三须

清

银质

长 36 厘米，重 48.8 克

Silver Whisker-like Tools of Three Pieces

Qing Dynasty

Silver

Length 36 cm/ Weight 48.8 g

环形链，一头有两猴雕刻，带一钟、一铃、
一花篮。底端坠有小镊子、掏耳勺、剔牙棒
各一件。卫生器具，完整无损。

陕西医史博物馆藏

The chain is annular-looped. The design of two
monkeys is carved on one end of the chain.
It also has the designs of a ball-shaped bell,
a jingle bell and a gaily decorated basket. A
tweezer, an ear pick and a toothpick are hung
at the bottom.The chain was used as a sanitary
tool. It is intact in shape.

Preserved in Shaanxi Museum of Medical History

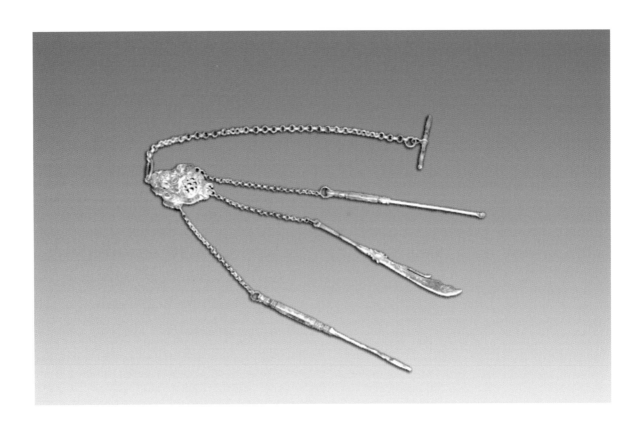

银三须

清

银质

长 34 厘米，重 28 克

Silver Whisker-like Tools of Three Pieces

Qing Dynasty

Silver

Length 34 cm/ Weight 28 g

环形链，链头带一长棒，有小刀、剔牙棒、掏耳勺。卫生器具。完整无损。

陕西医史博物馆藏

The chain is annular-looped. Its head has a long stick. The chain is connected with a knife, a tooth stick and an ear picker. It was used as a sanitary tool. The chain is intact in shape.

Preserved in Shaanxi Museum of Medical History

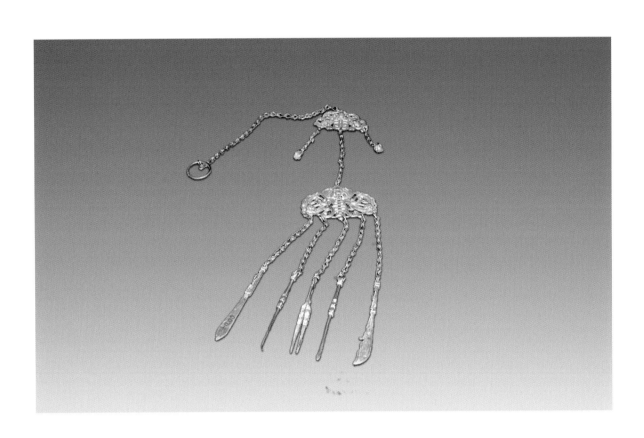

银五须

清

银质

长 46 厘米，重 61.5 克

Silver Whisker-like Tools of Five Pieces

Qing Dynasty

Silver

Length 46 cm/ Weight 61.5 g

环形链，有两个小铃，链中间有一"寿"字，带五须，坠有柳叶刀、剔牙棒、小镊子、掏耳勺、尖刀各一件。卫生器具。完整无损。

陕西医史博物馆藏

The chain is annular-looped and has two small bells. A character "Shou" (means longevity) is carved in the middle of the chain. It has 5 "whiskers" pendent with a lancet, a toothpick, a tweezer, an ear pick and a small knife used as a sanitary appliance. The chain is intact in shape.

Preserved in Shaanxi Museum of Medical History

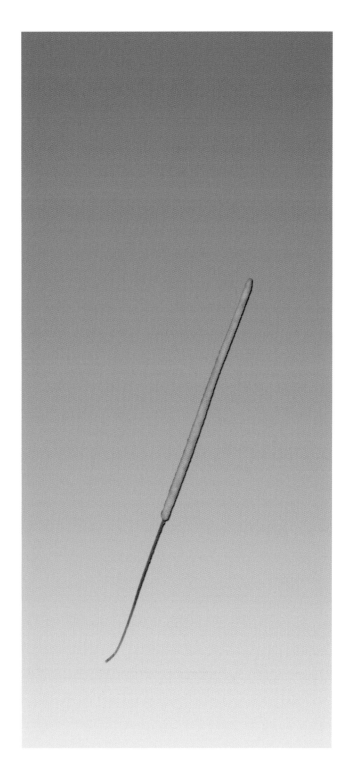

清理耳鼻工具

清

骨柄钢针

通长 17.6 厘米，柄径 0.3 厘米

A Nose and Ear Cleaning Tool

Qing Dynasty

Bone Handel, Steel Needle

Length 17.6 cm/ Handle Diameter 0.3 cm

长形，为卫生用具。这是该馆通过自购收藏的清末理发用卫生工具之一。这种工具常用做清洁耳鼻内污物。保存基本完好。

中华医学会 / 上海中医药大学医史博物馆藏

The tool is long in shape and was often used by hairdressers as a sanitary tool for cleaning customers' ears and noses. It was made in the late Qing Dynasty. The relic was purchased by the museum. The relic is basically well preserved.

Preserved in Chinese Medical Association/ Museum of Chinese Medicine, Shanghai University of Traditional Chinese Medicine

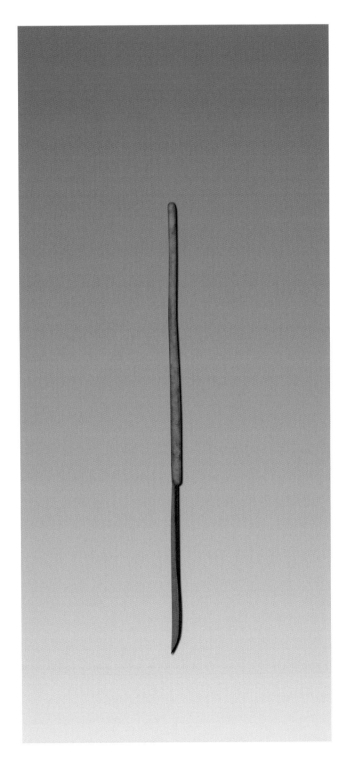

清理耳鼻工具

清

骨柄钢针

通长 17.6 厘米，柄径 0.3 厘米

A Nose and Ear Cleaning Tool

Qing Dynasty

Bone Handle, Steel Needle

Length 17.6 cm/ Handle diameter 0.3 cm

长形，为卫生用具。这是该馆通过自购收藏的清末理发用卫生工具之一。这种工具常用做清洁耳鼻内污物。保存基本完好。

中华医学会 / 上海中医药大学医史博物馆藏

The tool is long in shape and was often used by hairdressers as a sanitary tool for cleaning customers' ears and noses. It was made in the late Qing Dynasty. The relic was purchased by the museum. The relic is basically well preserved.

Preserved in Chinese Medical Association/ Museum of Chinese Medicine, Shanghai University of Traditional Chinese Medicine

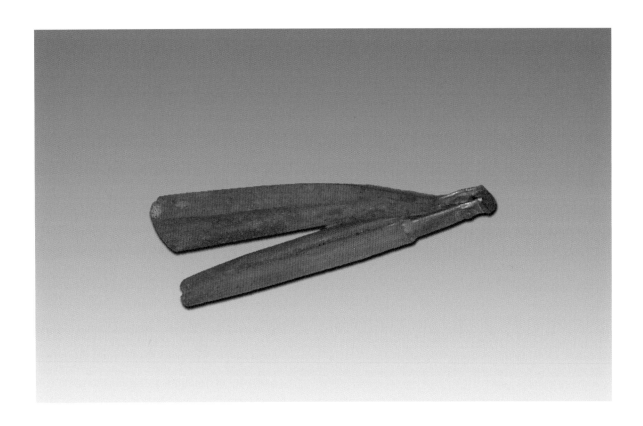

剃刀

清

铁刀木柄

通长 21.4 厘米，宽 2.4 厘米，刃长 6.6 厘米

Shaver

Qing Dynasty

Iron Knife, Wood Handle

Length 21.4 cm/ Width 2.4 cm/ Edge Length 6.6 cm

刀形，为刀具。该藏铁刀木柄，可折叠，有使用痕迹。1958 年入藏。保存基本完好。

中华医学会 / 上海中医药大学医史博物馆藏

The knife-shaped tool was used as a shaver. It has an iron-made knife and a wood-made handle. It is foldable and shows signs of use. The relic was collected by the museum in 1958. The relic is basically well preserved.

Preserved in Chinese Medical Association/ Museum of Chinese Medicine, Shanghai University of Traditional Chinese Medicine

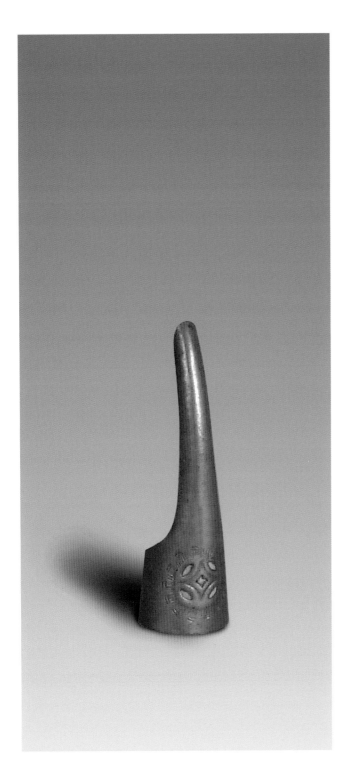

指甲套

清

铜质

长 5.1 厘米，宽 1.55 厘米，厚 0.05 厘米

Fingernail Cover

Qing Dynasty

Copper

Length 5.1 cm/ Width 1.55 cm/ Thickness 0.05 cm

指甲形，为装饰品。该藏用铜片制成，表面光滑，工艺精细，上有镂空花卉图案。1959年入藏。保存基本完好。

中华医学会 / 上海中医药大学医史博物馆藏

The cover is in the shape of a fingernail and was used as an ornament. The relic was delicately made of a copper sheet, with smooth surface and hollowed-out flower patterns. The relic was collected by the museum in 1959. The relic is basically well preserved.

Preserved in Chinese Medical Association/ Museum of Chinese Medicine, Shanghai University of Traditional Chinese Medicine

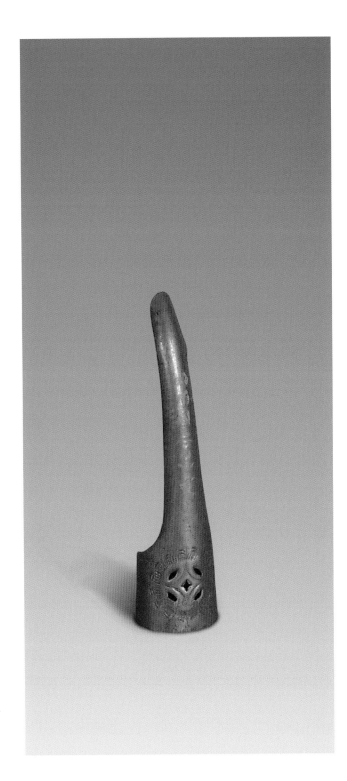

指甲套

清

铜质

长 6.4 厘米，宽 1.7 厘米，厚 0.05 厘米

Fingernail Cover

Qing Dynasty

Copper

Length 6.4 cm/ Width 1.7 cm/ Thickness 0.05 cm

指甲形，为装饰品。该藏用铜片制成，表面
光滑，工艺精细，上有镂空花卉图案。1959
年入藏。保存基本完好。

中华医学会／上海中医药大学医史博物馆藏

The cover is in the shape of a fingernail and was
used as an ornament. The relic was delicately
made of a copper sheet, with a smooth surface
and hollowed-out flower patterns. The relic was
collected by the museum in 1959. The relic is
basically well preserved.

Preserved in Chinese Medical Association/
Museum of Chinese Medicine, Shanghai
University of Traditional Chinese Medicine

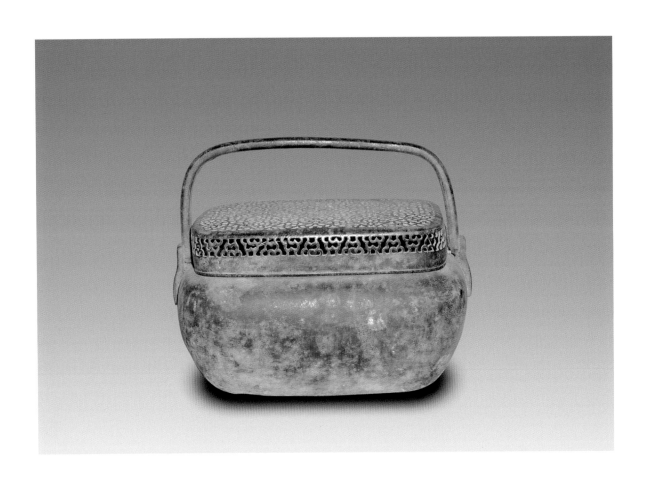

铜手炉

清

铜质

长 18 厘米，高 12.5 厘米，底径 17 厘米，重 1550 克

Copper Handwarmer

Qing Dynasty

Copper

Length 18 cm/ Height 12.5 cm/ Bottom Diameter 17 cm/ Weight 1,550 g

子母口，四棱鼓腹，圈足上带一手柄，有盖，

盖为缠枝网盖。生活器具。完整无损。

陕西医史博物馆藏

The handwarmer has a snap-lid, a swelling belly with four ridges, and a ring foot connected with a handle. The cover is decorated with entangled floral branch design. The relic was used as an appliance for daily purpose. The relic is intact in shape.

Preserved in Shaanxi Museum of Medical History

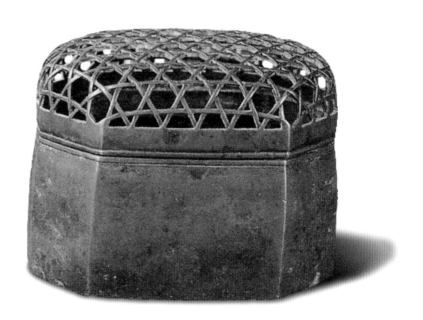

八角铜手炉

清

铜质

长 12.5 厘米，宽 7.8 厘米，高 9.2 厘米

用于取暖、保温。

上海中医药博物馆藏

Octagon Copper Handwarmer

Qing Dynasty

Copper

Length 12.5 cm/ Width 7.8 cm/ Height 9.2 cm

The handwarmer was used for keeping warm.

Preserved in Shanghai Museum of Traditional Chinese Medicine

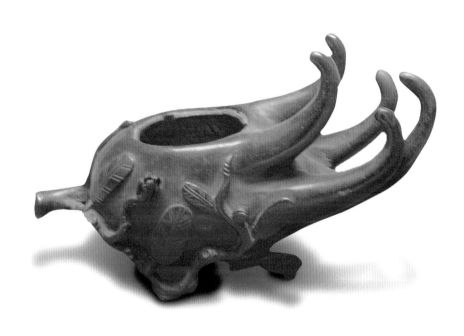

佛手

清

铜质

长 25 厘米，宽 9 厘米

做成佛手状的熏炉，惜盖已失。由上海文物商店征集。

成都中医药大学中医药传统文化博物馆藏

Censer in the Shape of Fingered Citron

Qing Dynasty

Copper

Length 25 cm/ Width 9 cm

The relic is a censer in the shape of the fingered Citron (its Chinese name means Buddha's hand). The cover was lost. It was collected from a Shanghai antique shop.

Preserved in Museum of Traditional Chinese Medicine Culture, Chengdu University of Traditional Chinese Medicine

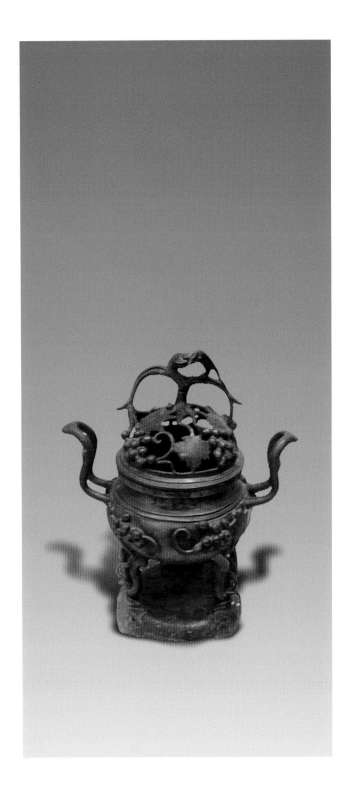

熏炉

清

铜质

高 37.5 厘米

Censer

Qing Dynasty

Copper

Height 37.5 cm

炉身为圆鼓形，束颈，顶平口，与盖和底座通过堆塑葡萄纹，形成一个整体，松鼠形钮，环形双耳。器物构思精巧，一气呵成，几部分比例协调，大小适中，具有典型的东方气质。由四川省文物商店征集。

成都中医药大学中医药传统文化博物馆藏

The censer body is in the shape of a round drum. It has a restricted neck and a flat mouth. The mouth is connected to the censer cover and pedestal with paste-on-paste grapes decorations to form an integrated body. The censer has a squirrel-shaped knob and a pair of annular ears. The relic was delicately designed and bears a classic oriental style. The components are in suitable proportion and size. The censer was collected from a Sichuan antique shop.

Preserved in Museum of Traditional Chinese Medicine Culture, Chengdu University of Traditional Chinese Medicine

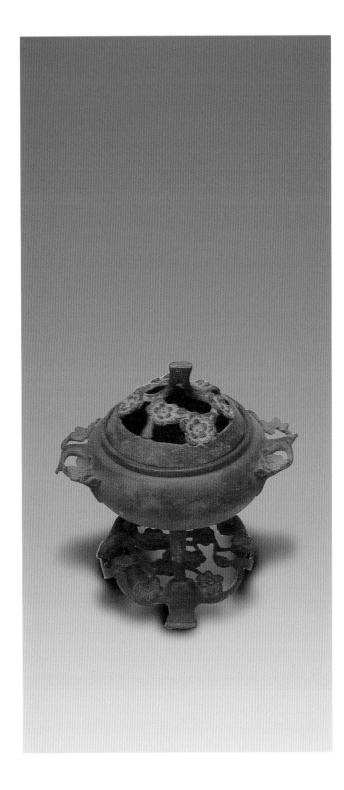

熏炉

清

铜质

宽 16.5 厘米，炉径 9.7 厘米，底径 10.2 厘米

底座：高 2.4 厘米

盖：高 4.5 厘米

Censer

Qing Dynasty

Copper

Width 16.5 cm/ Body Diameter 9.7 cm/ Bottom

Diameter 10.2 cm

Pedestal: Height 2.4 cm

Cover: Height 4.5 cm

器形完整，做工精美。炉身为圆鼓形，弧形底，柱形三足，堆塑梅花形双耳，底座为梅枝盘绕而成，上面点缀朵朵梅花，盖也呈梅树枝形，有梅花点缀其间，梅枝间的空隙即为香烟出口，盖上有人字形钮。从天津文物商店征集。

成都中医药大学中医药传统文化博物馆藏

The relic is intact in shape and is delicately made. The censer body is in the shape of a round drum. It has an arc-shaped pedestal, with three pillar-like feet. The body has two ears in the shape of plum blossoms. The pedestal is formed by entangled plum flower branches, decorated on its surface with plum blossoms. The cover is also adorned with plum flower branch patterns, embellished with plum flowers. The interspace of the plum branches serves as ventilating incense. The cover is equipped with a knob bearing resemblance to the character "人". The relic was collected form a Tianjin antique shop.

Preserved in Museum of Traditional Chinese Medicine Culture, Chengdu University of Traditional Chinese Medicine

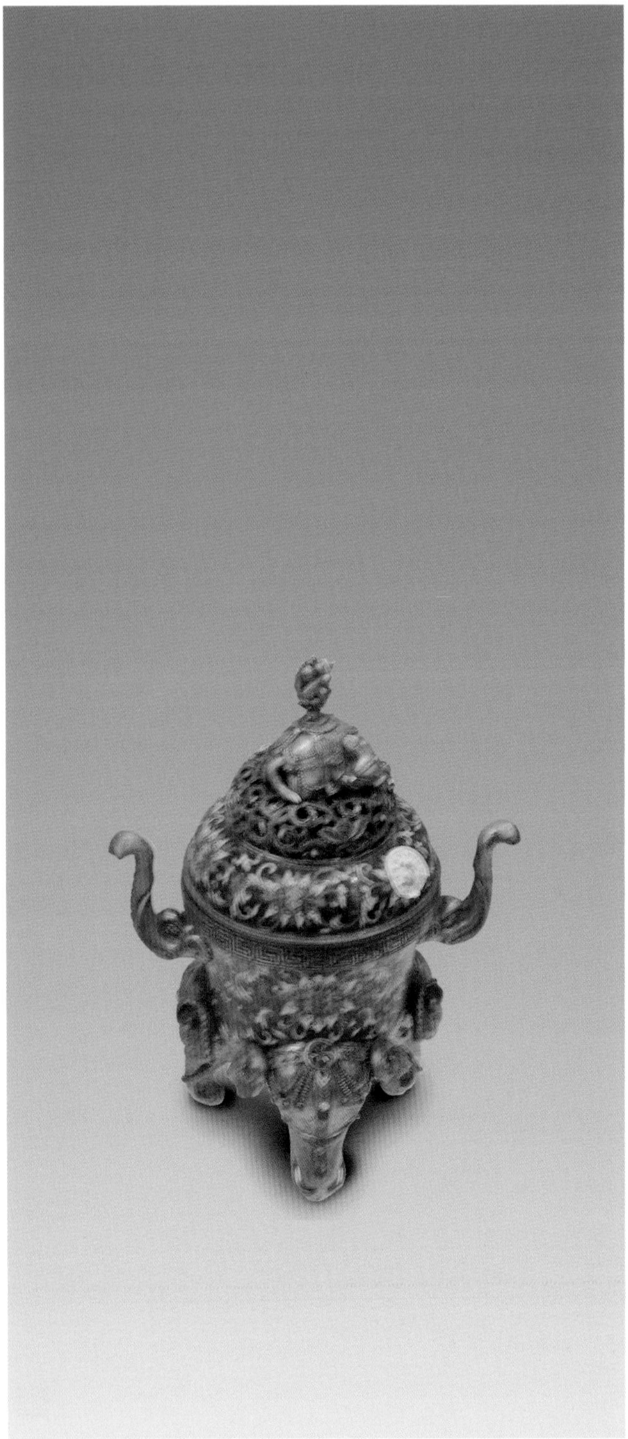

熏炉

清

铜质

高 42 厘米

Censer

Qing Dynasty

Copper

Height 42 cm

景泰蓝制作，象鼻形三足，双耳，盖上塑动
物形装饰，器身上有钻石镶嵌。由四川省文
物拍卖公司征集。

成都中医药大学中医药传统文化博物馆藏

The censer was made of cloisonne. It has three
feet in the shape of elephant trunks. The cover
is decorated with animal-shaped patterns. The
body is inlaid with diamonds. The relic was
collected from a relics auction company in
Sichuan.

Preserved in Chinese Medical Association/
Museum of Chinese Medicine, Shanghai
University of Traditional Chinese Medicine

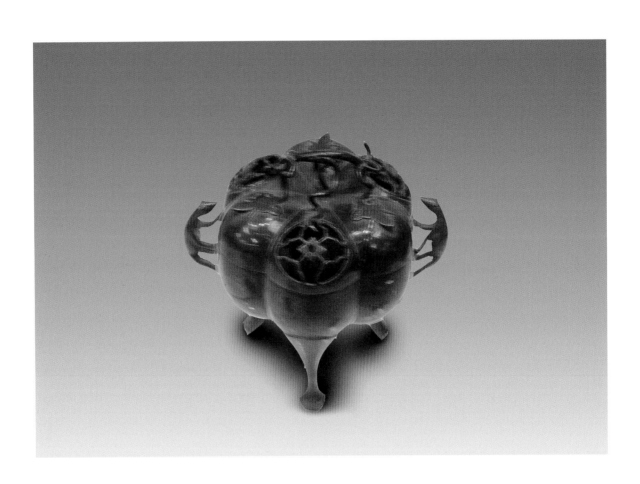

熏炉

清

铜质

腹径 10.4 厘米，高 13 厘米

Censer

Qing Dynasty

Copper

Belly Diameter 10.4 cm/ Height 13 cm

构思巧妙，做工精湛，保存完好，具有较高的艺术价值。器物比例匀称，炉身为瓜棱形，弧形底，蹄形三足，兽形双耳，盖有子母口与身相合，由三组缠枝纹镂空形成香烟出口。兽形纽。整个器物呈黑古漆色，造型一气呵成，简洁明快，令人回味。上海文物商店征集。

成都中医药大学中医药传统文化博物馆藏

The censer was delicately designed, finely made and well preserved. It is of high artistic value. The well-proportioned censer body bears resemblance to a melon with ridges. The censer has an arc-shaped bottom, three hoof-like feet, two beast ears, a snap-lid and an animal-shaped knob. The censer is decorated with three groups of hollowed twined branch patterns for the purpose of ventilating incense. The censer was lacquered with vintage black paint and the style is smooth and simplicity. The relic was collected from a Shanghai antique.

Preserved in Chinese Medical Association/ Museum of Chinese Medicine, Shanghai University of Traditional Chinese Medicine

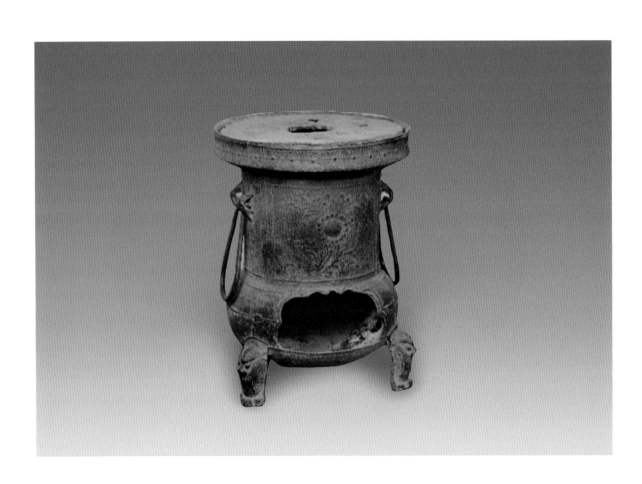

炼丹炉

清

合金

腹径 32 厘米，通高 69 厘米

Alchemy Furnace

Qing Dynasty

Alloy

Belly Diameter 32 cm/ Height 69 cm

炉盘四周刻有四瓣花纹，圆桶形炉体，左、右各有两个桥形钮，U 形双环，鼓状炉底，三兽足。炉体有草药花纹。古时用来炼制丹药的工具。

北京御生堂中医药博物馆藏

The furnace, which is shaped like a cylinder, has two bridge-shaped knobs, double U-shaped rings, a drum-shaped base and three beast feet. The furnace tray is carved with four-petal flowers and the furnace body is engraved with the herbs motifs. It was used for alchemy. Preserved in Chinese Medicine Museum of Beijing Yu Sheng Tang Drugstore

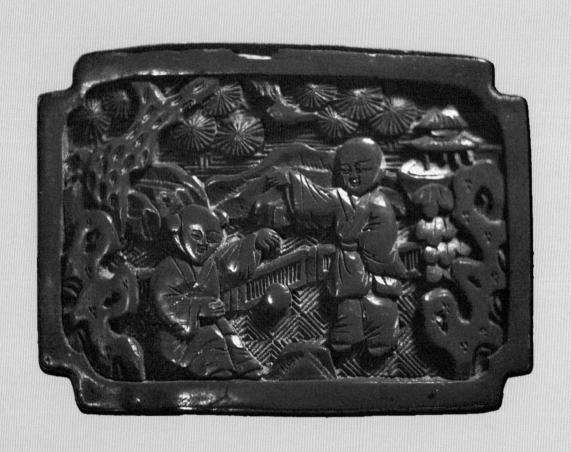

蹴鞠图漆绘铜牌

清

铜质

长 8.5 厘米，宽 4.5 厘米

铜牌表面施红漆，长方形，四角微凹。图案饰于牌的正面，为二童子做蹴鞠游戏状，背景松树、楼阁掩映，别具情致。

中国体育博物馆藏

Lacquered Bronze Plate with Cuju Painting

Qing Dynasty

Copper

Length 8.5 cm/ Width 4.5 cm

The plate surface is lacquered with red paint. It is rectangle in shape, with four slightly dented corners. The front side of the plate is decorated with a painting which depicts two kids playing the game of Cuju (an ancient Chinese ball game). The backdrop of the painting consists of pine trees and pavilions. The relic gives out a unique feeling of delight.

Preserved in China Sports Museum

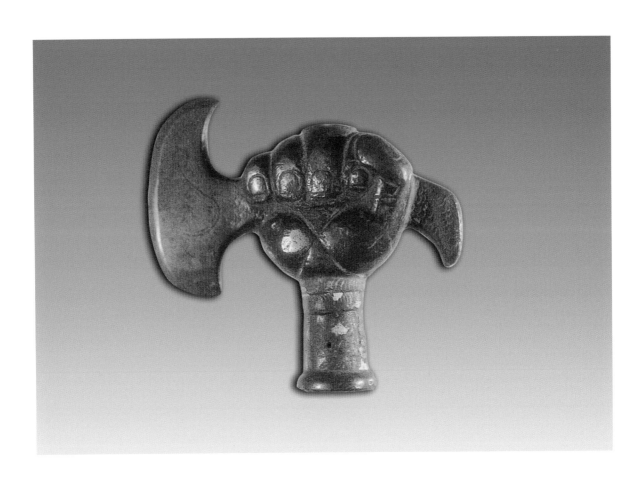

手柄铜斧

清

铜质

宽 15 厘米，高 13 厘米

Copper Axe with Handle

Qing Dynasty

Copper

Width 15 cm/ Height 13 cm

为古代武术中的一种砍劈器械。斧为弧刃，柄端呈手的形状握住弧刃，斧下有銎，可以穿长木柄。

中国体育博物馆藏

The axe was used as a hacking tool in ancient martial arts. The axe has an arc-shaped cutting edge and a hand-shaped handle with a gesture of holding the axe. There is a hole on the axe for installing a long wood handle.

Preserved in China Sports Museum

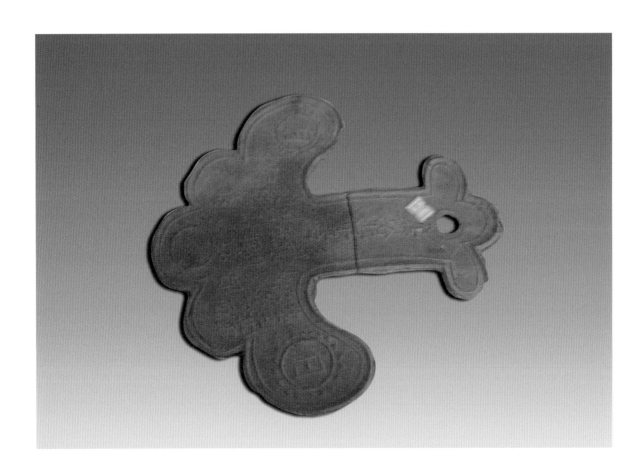

铁云牌

清

铁质

长 44 厘米，高 45 厘米，重 4300 克

Iron "Yun-pai"

Qing Dynasty

Iron

Length 44 cm/ Height 45 cm/ Weight 4,300 g

云状，上有铭文"光绪十七年主造"。宗教乐
器，有残。陕西省眉县太白山征集。

陕西医史博物馆藏

"Yun-pai" was a religious musical instrument.
The relic bears resemblance to the shape of
clouds. The body is inscribed with an inscription
"Guang Xu Shi Qi Nian Zhu Zao" (made in the
17th year of Emperor Guangxu's reign). It is not
complete and was collected in Taibai Mountain,
Meixian County, Shaanxi Province.

Preserved in Shaanxi Museum of Medical History

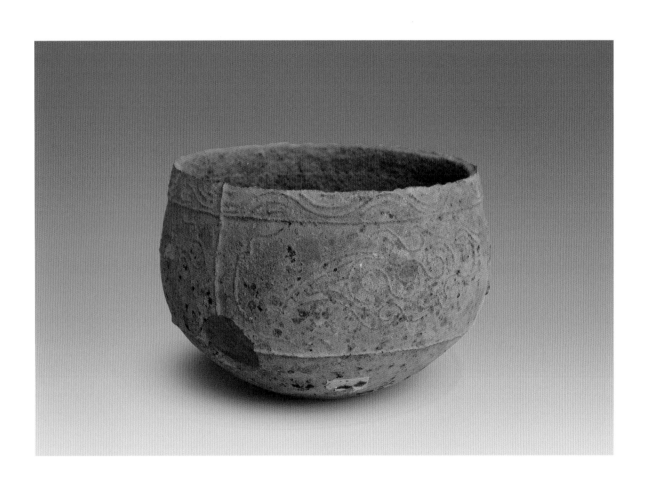

铁磬

清

铁质

口径 24.5 厘米，高 19 厘米，重 7000 克

Iron "Qing"

Qing Dynasty

Iron

Mouth Diameter 24.5 cm/ Height 19 cm/ Weight 7,000 g

圆口，圆腹，圆底，下腹和底之间有三圆孔，

有铭文"道光十年造"。佛教乐器，完整无损。

陕西医史博物馆藏

"Qing" was a Buddhist musical instrument. The relic has a round mouth, a round belly and a round bottom. There are three holes between the lower belly and the bottom. There is an inscription "Dao Guang Shi Nian Zao" (which means "made in the 10th year of Emperor Daoguang's reign"). The relic is intact.

Preserved in Shaanxi Museum of Medical History

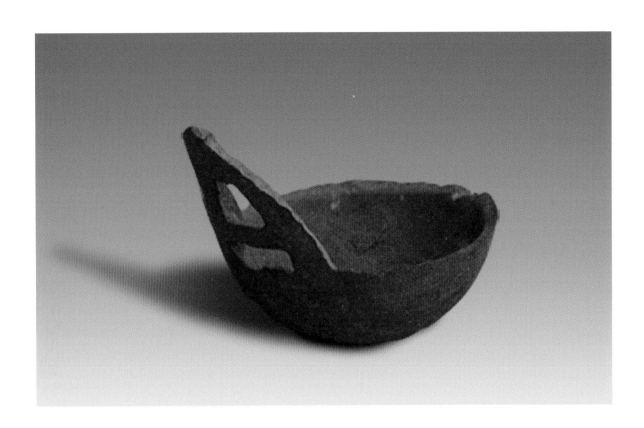

铁灯

清

铁质

口径 8 厘米，通高 8 厘米，重 250 克

Iron Lamp

Qing Dynasty

Iron

Mouth Diameter 8 cm/ Height 8 cm/ Weight 250 g

半球形灯碗,后侧沿有一半圆加十字形装饰。
生活器具。完整无损。

陕西医史博物馆藏

The lamp bowls is hemispheric in shape. A cross-like decoration with a semi-circle design is added to the posterior rim. The lamp was used for daily life purposes. The relic is intact in shape.

Preserved in Shaanxi Museum of Medical History

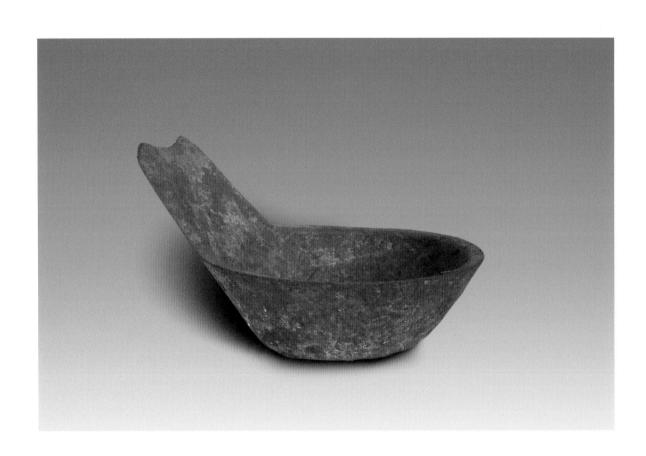

油灯盏

清

铁质

宽 15 厘米，通高 8.5 厘米

Oil Lamp

Qing Dynasty

Iron

Width 15 cm/ Height 8.5 cm

勺状，灯具。该藏生铁铸造，工艺粗糙，平底，
有使用痕迹。1959 年入藏。保存基本完好，
锈蚀较重。

　中华医学会 / 上海中医药大学医史博物馆藏

The lamp is in the shape of a ladle and it
was used for lighting purpose. The lamp was
roughly made of pig iron. It has a flattened
bottom with signs of use. It was collected in the
year of 1959. It is basically well preserved with
relatively severe rusting.

Preserved in Chinese Medical Association/
Museum of Chinese Medicine, Shanghai
University of Traditional Chinese Medicine

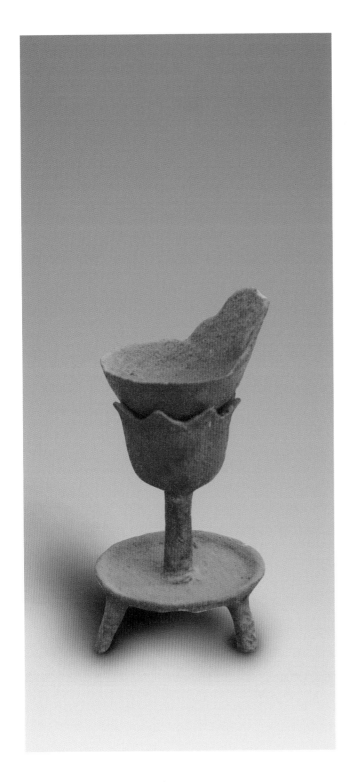

铁灯

清

铁质

通高 18.6 厘米，重 8500 克

Iron Lamp

Qing Dynasty

Iron

Height 18.6 cm/ Weight 8,500 g

灯碗呈勺状，中间为一杯状，底座为圆盘三
足。生活器具。完整无损。陕西省乾县征集。

陕西医史博物馆藏

The lamp bowl is in the shape of a ladle. The
mid-section of the lamp is like a cup. The
pedestal consist of a round plate and three feet.
It was used for daily life purposes. It is intact
in shape and was collected in Qianxian County,
Shaanxi Province.

Preserved in Shaanxi Museum of Medical History

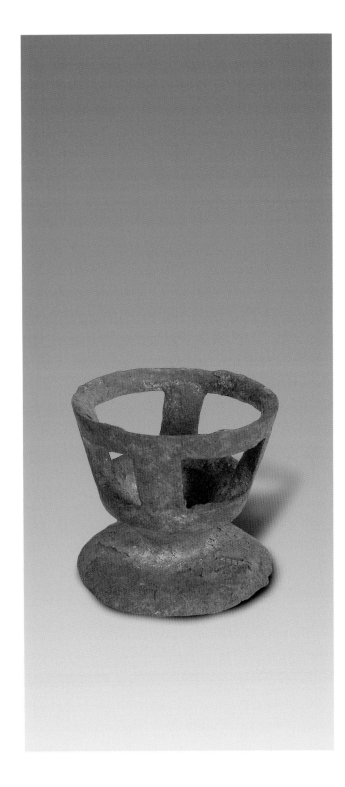

油灯盏座

清

铁质

宽 9.7 厘米，通高 8.2 厘米

Oil Lamp Pedestal

Qing Dynasty

Iron

Width 9.7 cm/ Height 8.2 cm

灯座。该藏生铁铸造，工艺粗糙，平底，有

使用痕迹。1954 年入藏。保存基本完好。

　中华医学会 / 上海中医药大学医史博物馆藏

The lamp pedestal was roughly made of pig
iron. It has a flattened bottom with signs of
use. It was collected in the year of 1954. It is
basically well preserved.

Preserved in Chinese Medical Association/
Museum of Chinese Medicine, Shanghai
University of Traditional Chinese Medicine

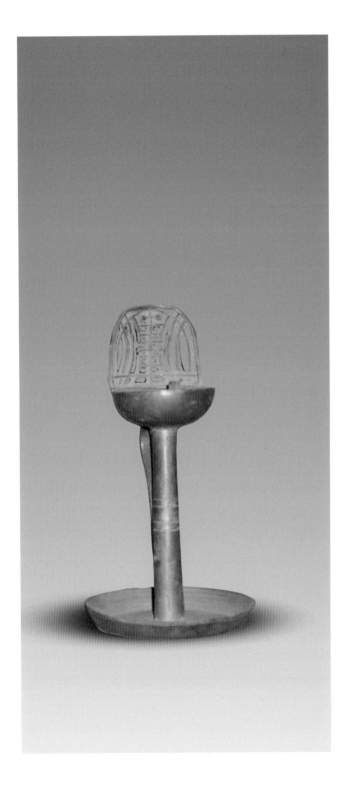

铜灯

清

铜质

口径 6.5 厘米，底径 9.5 厘米，通高 20 厘米，重 350 克

Copper Lamp

Qing Dynasty

Copper

Mouth Diameter 6.5 cm/ Bottom Diameter 9.5 cm/ Height 20 cm/ Weight 350 g

灯呈豆状，灯碗内有灯眼，口沿上有"萬"字造型，灯杆有一耳形手柄，底座为盘状。生活器具。完整无损。

陕西医史博物馆藏

The lamp is in the shape of a bean. The lampwick is inside the lamp bowl. On the mouth rim there is a design in resemblance to character "萬". The lamp pole has an ear-shaped handle. The pedestal is like a plate. The lamp was used for daily life purposes. It is intact in shape.

Preserved in Shaanxi Museum of Medical History

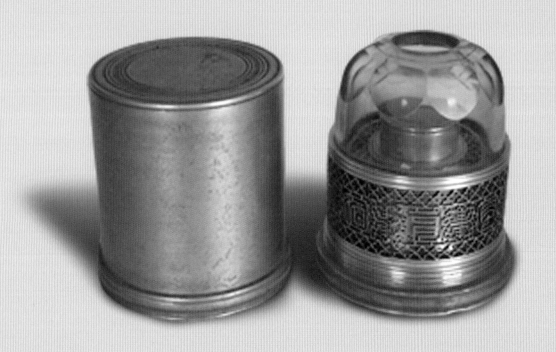

铜油灯

清

铜质

外径 7.7 厘米，通高 8.95 厘米

圆柱状，灯具。该藏由铜盖罩、铜油壶、铜灯芯冒、玻璃罩等组成，灯座与罩由螺口连接，工艺精细，造型美观，底部有"增顺"押记。1955 年入藏。保存完好。

中华医学会 / 上海中医药大学医史博物馆藏

Copper Oil Lamp

Qing Dynasty

Copper

Outer Diameter 7.7 cm/ Height 8.95 cm

The lamp is cylindrical in shape. The whole set consists of a copper cover, a copper oiler, a cooper lampwick cover, and a glass cover. The lamp pedestal is connected by a cover and a screw opening. The lamp was delicately made and designed. The bottom has a charge sign "Zeng Shun". The relic was collected in 1955. It is well preserved.

Preserved in Chinese Medical Association/Museum of Chinese Medicine, Shanghai University of Traditional Chinese Medicine

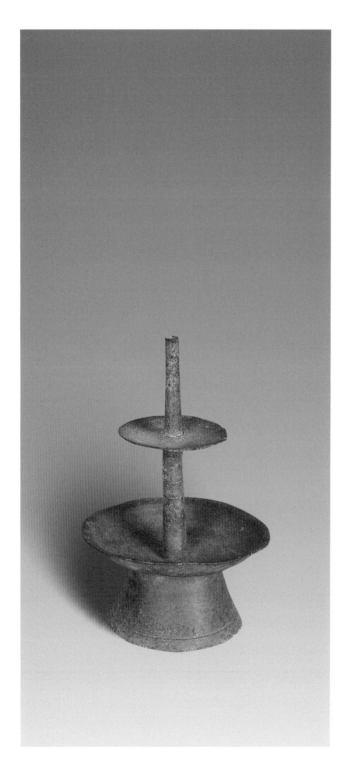

铝台灯

清

铝质

宽 8.95 厘米，通高 13.7 厘米

Aluminum Table Lamp

Qing Dynasty

Aluminum

Width 8.95 cm/ Height 13.7 cm

灯盏状，灯具。该藏工艺一般，圈足，分上、

下两层，有使用痕迹。1983 年入藏。保存基

本完好。

中华医学会 / 上海中医药大学医史博物馆藏

The workmanship of the lamp is ordinary. It
has a ring foot and is composed of an upper
and a lower parts. The lamp shows signs of use.
It was collected in 1983 and is basically well
preserved.

Preserved in Chinese Medical Association/
Museum of Chinese Medicine, Shanghai
University of Traditional Chinese Medicine

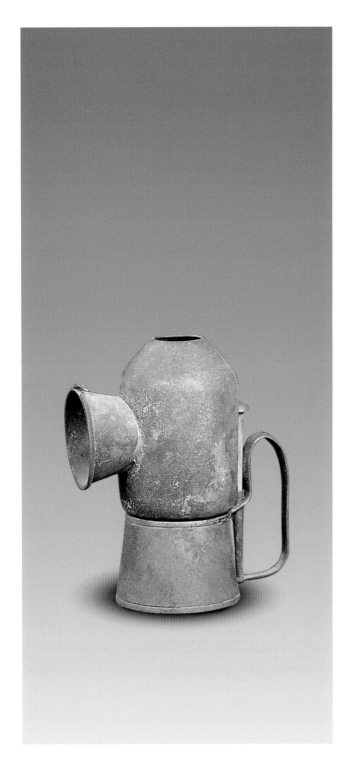

铜灭蚊灯

清

铜质

上口径 2.5 厘米，底径 6.5 厘米，通高 12 厘米

喇叭口：内口径 3 厘米，外口径 4.5 厘米

Copper Mosquito-Killing Lamp

Qing Dynasty

Copper

Upper Mouth Diameter 2.5 cm/ Bottom Diameter

6.5 cm/ Height 12 cm

Trumped-like Mouth: Inner Diameter 3 cm/ Outer

Diameter 4.5 cm

分上、下两节。上节有口，腹有喇叭口，用
于透光，使蚊子被吸入；下节为油灯。上、
下节相交处有子母口。

上海中医药博物馆藏

The lamp is composed of an upper and a lower
sections. The upper part has a mouth, and the
belly has a trumped-like mouth. The upper
section gives out light to attract mosquitoes and
the lower section is an oil lamp. The two parts
are connected with a snap-lid.

Preserved in Shanghai Museum of Traditional
Chinese Medicine

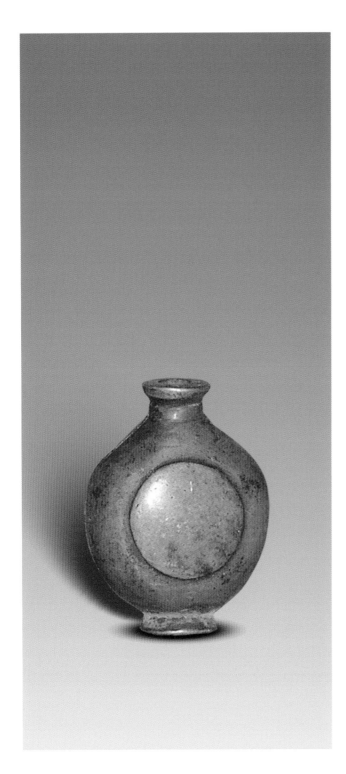

铜鼻烟壶

清

铜质

口径 1.5 厘米，底径 1.5 厘米，通高 5 厘米，

重 50 克

Copper Snuff Bottle

Qing Dynasty

Copper

Mouth Diameter 1.5 cm/ Bottom Diameter

1.5 cm/ Height 5 cm/ Weight 50 g

小喇叭平口，圆腹，平底，腹上有一圆棱。

烟具。完整无损。

陕西医史博物馆藏

The snuff bottle has a small trumpet-like flattened mouth, a round belly and a flattened bottom. The belly is decorated with a protruding round ridge. The snuff bottle was used as a smoking tool. It is intact in shape.

Preserved in Shaanxi Museum of Medical History

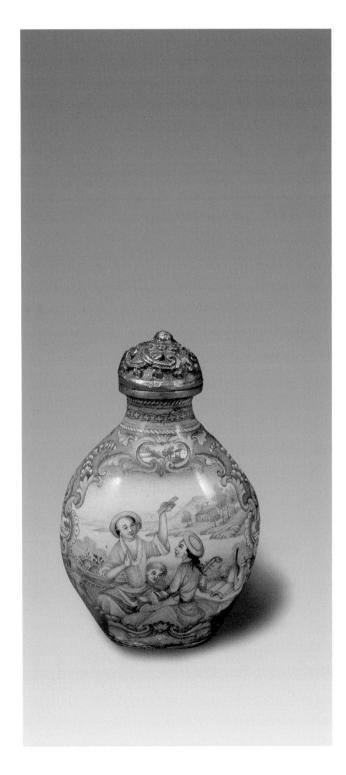

画珐琅人物纹烟壶

清

铜质鎏金

口径 1.6 厘米，足径 2 厘米，通高 6.3 厘米

Snuff Bottle with Enamel Figure Painting

Qing Dynasty

Gold-decorated Copper

Mouth Diameter 1.6 cm/ Bottom Diameter 2 cm/ Height 6.3 cm

铜胎。圆口，扁腹，圈足，盖面隆起，附象牙勺。口、盖、足鎏金。腹、背两面开光，绘洋人戏狗或执乐器边歌边舞，以山水为背景。足内有蓝彩楷书"大清乾隆年制"官窑款。

山东省文物总店藏

The snuff bottle was made from a copper mold. It has a round mouth, a flattened belly and a ring foot. The cover surface protrudes upward and is equipped with an ivory spoon. The mouth, cover and foot are all gilded with gold. The belly and back are decorated with paintings depicting foreigners playing with dogs or singing and dancing with musical instruments, with mountains and waters as backdrops. On the bottom there goes an inscription written in blue regular script reading "Da Qing Qian Long Nian Zhi" (meaning "made during the reign of Emperor Qianlong of the Qing Dynasty"), which proves that the relic was a product from an official ware.

Preserved in Shandong Antique Store

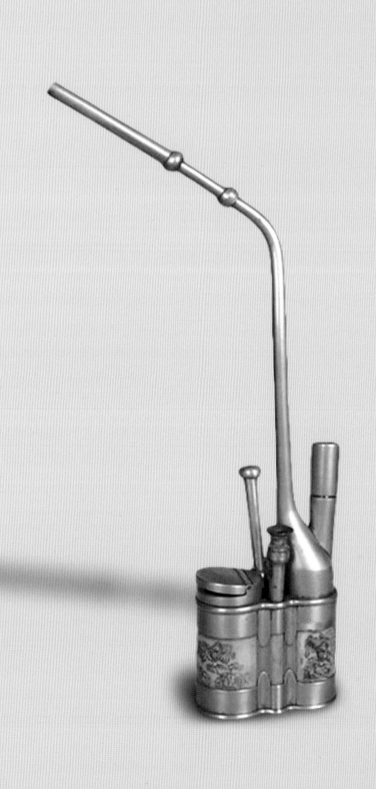

水烟筒

清

铜质

烟筒宽 6.6 厘米，厚 3.1 厘米，通高 29.5 厘米

烟筒形，烟具。该藏为铜制成，加工精细，烟筒表
面有花卉牙雕镶嵌。1955 年入藏。

中华医学会 / 上海中医药大学医史博物馆藏

Chinese Water Pipe

Qing Dynasty

Copper

Smoke Pipe 6.6 cm/ Thickness 3.1 cm/ Height 29.5 cm
The water pipe was used for smoking. It is made of
cooper and the craftsmanship is delicate. The surface
of the smoke pipe is inlaid with ivory carving along
with flower patterns. The relic was collected in 1955.
Preserved in Chinese Medical Association/Museum of
Chinese Medicine, Shanghai University of Traditional
Chinese Medicine

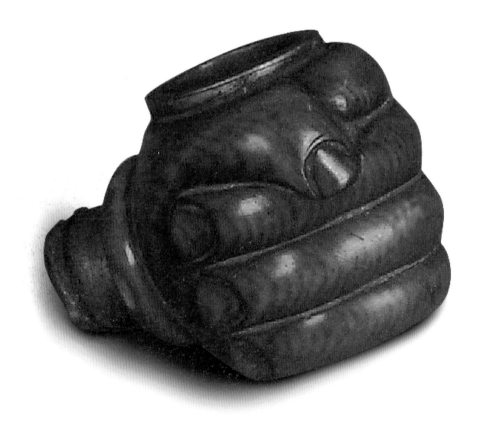

烟枪头

清

象牙、铜质

长 5.4 厘米，高 3.9 厘米

烟锅：口内径 1.9 厘米，口外径 2.45 厘米

烟锅状，医用。该藏用铜做烟锅及连管芯，镶嵌于象牙之中，象牙雕刻成人握手状。造型美观，雕工细腻，表面光滑，手感极好，烟锅外底刻有寿字图案。1959 年入藏。保存基本完好。

中华医学会 / 上海中医药大学医史博物馆藏

Smoking Pipe Head

Qing Dynasty

Ivory and Copper

Length 5.4 cm/ Height 3.9 cm

Smoke Pan: Inner Diameter 1.9 cm/ Outer Diameter 2.45 cm

The smoking pipe head is in the shape of a smoke pan and was used in medical settings. The smoke pan and the inner part of connecting pipe were made of copper, both of which are inlaid with ivory. The ivory is carved into the shape of a clenched hand. The style is beautiful and the carving craft is delicate. The surface feels smooth. There is a pattern in resemblance to the character "Shou" (longevity) at the bottom outside the smoke pan. The relic was collected in 1959. It is basically well preserved.

Preserved in Chinese Medical Association/Museum of Chinese Medicine, Shanghai University of Traditional Chinese Medicine

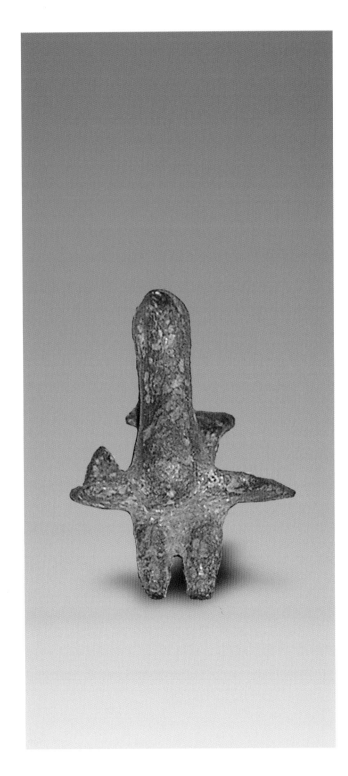

小铜鸽子像

清

铜质

口径 4 厘米，底径 1 厘米，通高 4.5 厘米，

重 50 克

Small Copper Pigeon

Qing Dynasty

Copper

Mouth Diameter 4 cm/ Bottom Diameter 1 cm/

Height 4.5 cm/ Weight 50 g

饰品。鸽子呈展翅飞翔状。完整无损。

陕西医史博物馆藏

The pigeon is an ornament. It presents like spreading its wings to fly. It is intact in shape.

Preserved in Shaanxi Museum of Medical History

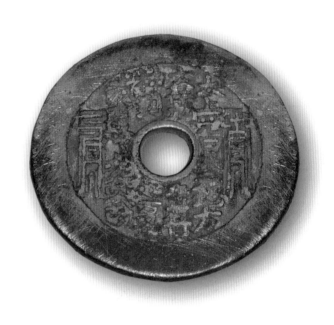

铜币

清

铜质

直径 4.6 厘米，重 50 克

上有铭文"太上咒日天元地方……"字样。完整无损。

陕西医史博物馆藏

Copper Coin

Qing Dynasty

Copper

Diameter 4.6 cm/ Weight 50 g

This copper coin is inscribed with Chinese characters reading "Tai Shang Zhou Ri Tian Yuan Di Fang…". It is intact in shape.

Preserved in Shaanxi Museum of Medical History

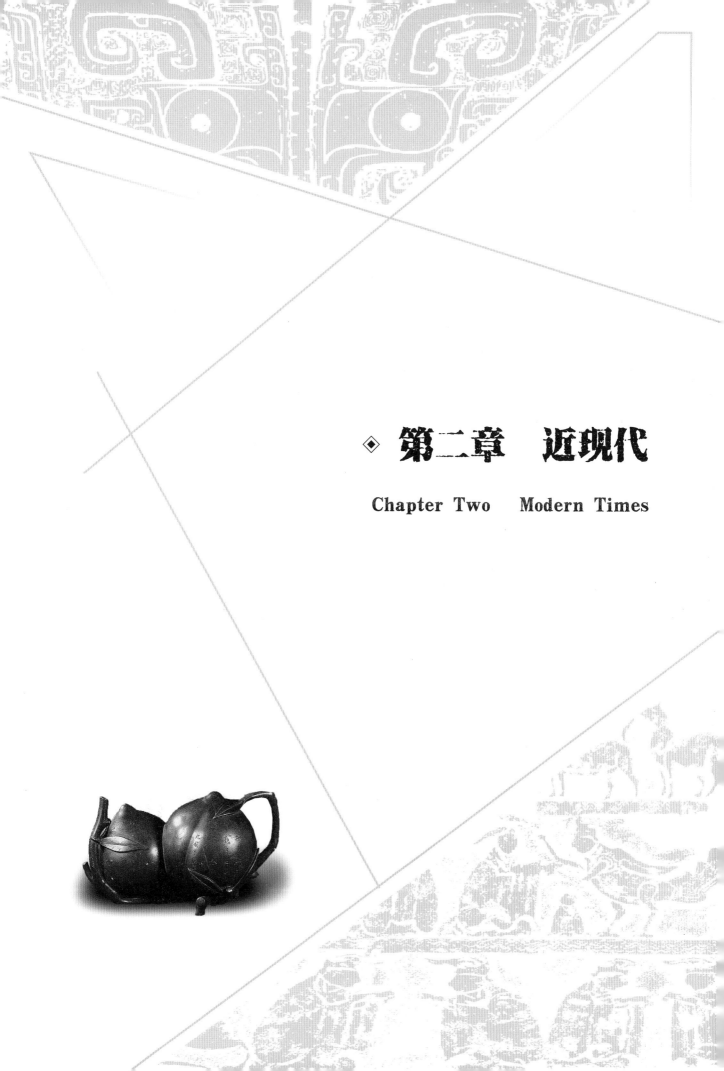

◈ 第二章　近现代

Chapter Two　Modern Times

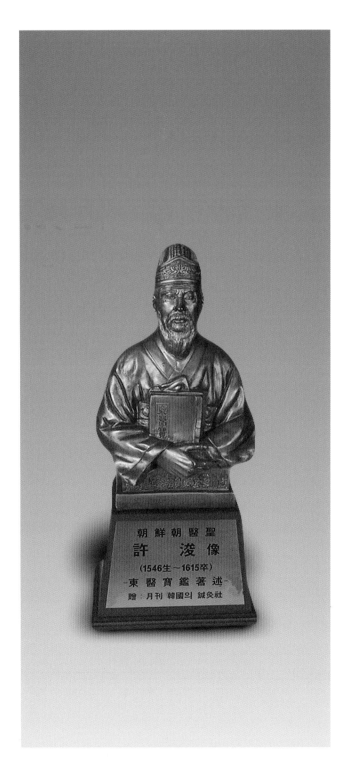

许浚像

民国时期

复合材料

宽 29.5 厘米，通高 71.5 厘米

Statue of Xu Jun

Republican Period

Composite Material

Width 29.5 cm/ Height 71.5 cm

半身人像，艺术品。该藏表面涂古铜色。为许浚双手捧《东医宝鉴》半身像，像正面下沿阳刻"医圣许浚像"。像之底座正面粘有铜铭牌，牌上书"朝鲜朝医圣 许浚像 赠 月刊 韩国 针灸社"等字样。许浚（1546—1615），朝鲜医家，著有《东医宝鉴》23卷，简明扼要地把中医介绍到朝鲜，被誉为"朝医圣"。保存基本完好。

中华医学会 / 上海中医药大学医史博物馆藏

The statue is an upper-body portraie and also an artwork. The statue is bronze-colored which described Xu Jun holding a book named *Dong Yi Bao Jian*. Under the statue, there are characters "Yi Sheng Xu Jun Xiang" (meaning "Xu Jun, Korean medical sage"), which are cut in relief. There is a copper nameplate on the surface of the base, on which there are characters recording the name and owner of the statue and so on. Xu Jun (1546–1615), a Korean traditional medical practitioner was the author of *Dong Yi Bao Jian* (Volume 23). He introduced Traditional Chinese Medicine to Korea briefly, and was honored as "Korean Medical Sage". The statue is basically well-preserved.

Preserved in Chinese Medical Association/Museum of Chinese Medicine, Shanghai University of Traditional Chinese Medicine

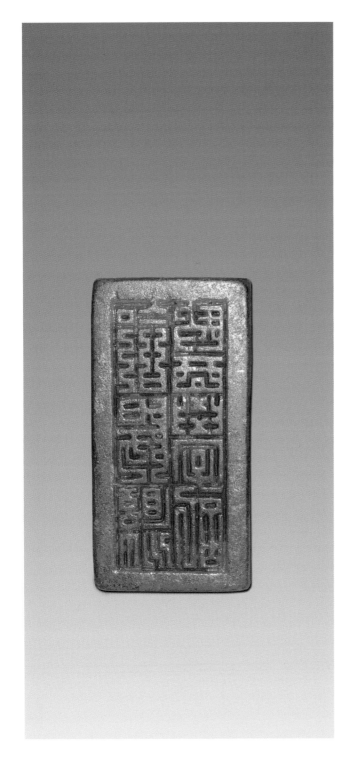

铜印（复制）

明

铜质

长8厘米，宽4厘米，高7.5厘米，重350克

Copper Seal (Copy)

Ming Dynasty

Copper

Length 8 cm/ Width 4 cm/ Height 7.5 cm/
Weight 350 g

印面呈长方形，"郃阳县医学记"印鉴，印背面有"礼部造，洪武三十五年十二月□日"，侧面"素字一千六十四号"字样。印鉴。完整无损。辽宁历史博物馆复制。

陕西医史博物馆藏

The surface of the seal is rectangular with characters which read "He Yang Xian Yi Xue Ji". There are characters on the back of the seal meaning "made by the Ministry of Rites on December (day ×), the 35th year of reign of Emperor Hongwu", as well as characters "Wen Zi No. 1064". The seal is well preserved. This one is the copy from Liaoning History Museum. Preserved in Shaanxi Museum of Medical History

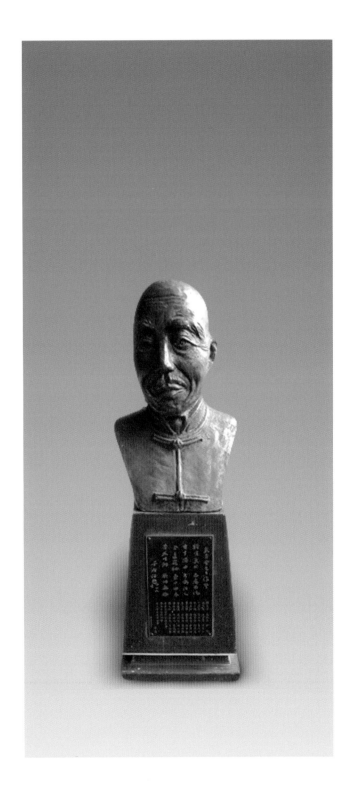

焦易堂半身铜像

近现代

铜质

宽 17 厘米，高 35 厘米

Half-Length Copper Statue of Jiao Yitang

Modern Times

Copper

Width 17 cm/ Height 35 cm

焦易堂，公元 1880—1950 年，讳希孟，字易堂，以字行，陕西武功县人。曾任中央国医馆馆长等。毕生为中医事业奔走呐喊，鞠躬尽瘁。1960 年，即纪念先生逝世十周年之际，由中医药学会（台湾地区）、香港中医师公会、台北市中医师公会等敬铸先生半身铜像一座，并刻有港台 30 位知名人士的姓名，捐赠给焦馆长的亲属。焦易堂馆长诞辰 120 周年之际，其子女将珍藏多年的焦易堂馆长铜像无偿捐赠给该馆陈列展览。

江苏省中医药博物馆藏

Jiao Yitang (1880–1950), also known as Xi Meng, had the courtesy name Yi Tang which was often used by him. He was from Wugong County, Shaanxi province. He was appointed as curator of Central Medical Hospital. He spent his lifetime for Chinese medical development. In 1960, namely the 10th anniversary of his death, the half-length statue of him was respectfully made by the Association of Chinese Medicine (Taiwan Area), the Hong Kong Chinese Herbalists Association, the Taipei Chinese Herbalists Association and so on. On the base inscribed names of over 30 celebrities from Hong Kong and Taiwan, who donated the statue to his relatives. In the year of his 120th birthday anniversary, his children donated the statue they preserved so many years to this museum.

Preserved in Jiangsu Museum of Traditional Chinese Medicine

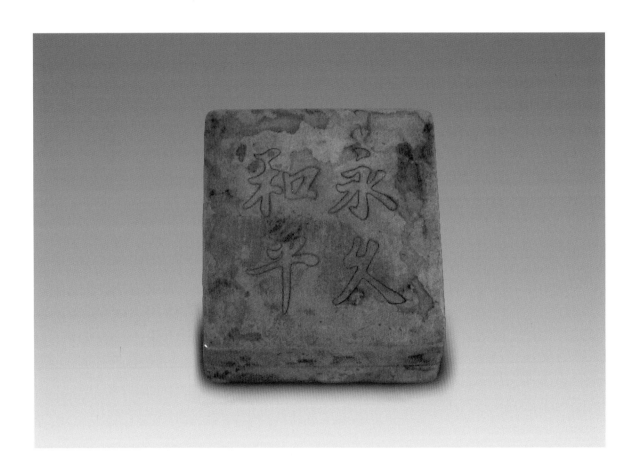

傅连暲墨盒

近现代

铜质

长 7.8 厘米，宽 7.8 厘米，厚 2.6 厘米

Fu Lianzhang's Ink Box

Modern Times

Copper

Length 7.8 cm/ Width 7.8 cm/ Thickness 2.6 cm

傅连暲，原名傅日新，福建长汀县人，医学家。中国人民解放军和新中国医疗卫生事业的奠基人、创始人之一。该藏为方盒形，由铜制成，盒盖浅刻"永久和平"，雕刻精细，表面光亮。文房用品。1991年入藏。

中华医学会 / 上海中医药大学医史博物馆藏

Fu Lianzhang, originally named Fu Rixin, was born in Changting County of Fujian Province. He is a medical scientist and one of the founders of the Chinese People's Liberation Army and Chinese health industry. The square box was made of copper, with four characters which read "Yong Jiu He Ping" (permanent peace) lightly engraved on the cover of the box. The box was finely carved with a brightness surface. It was one of the calligraphy supplies, and collected by the museum in 1991.

Preserved in Chinese Medical Association/ Museum of Chinese Medicine, Shanghai University of Traditional Chinese Medicine

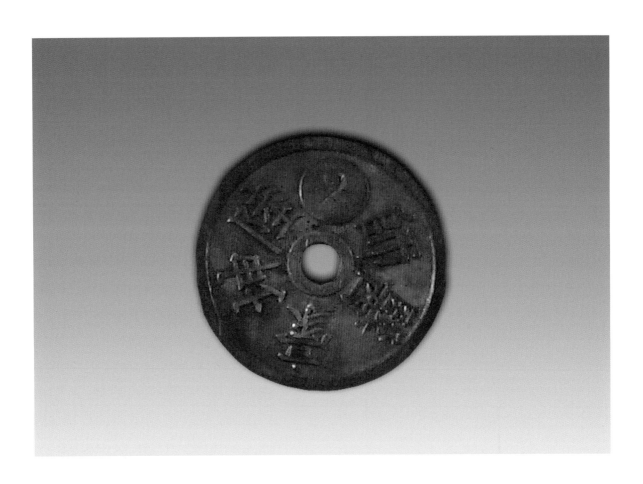

陆坤豪挂号牌

现代

铜质

直径 3 厘米，厚 0.1 厘米

Registration Tablet of Lu Kunhao

Modern Times

Copper

Diameter 3 cm/ Thickness 0.1 cm

圆形，为医事挂号牌。该藏用铜片制成，背面光滑，正面阳刻有"陆坤豪医师 2"字样，中心有圆孔。1955 年入藏。

中华医学会 / 上海中医药大学医史博物馆藏

The round tablet was made for medical registration. It was made of copper, with a smooth back and characters "Lu Kun Hao Yi Shi 2" meaning "Doctor Lu Kunhao 2" which was cut in relief on the surface. There is a hole in the middle. It was collected in 1955.

Preserved in Chinese Medical Association/ Museum of Chinese Medicine, Shanghai University of Traditional Chinese Medicine

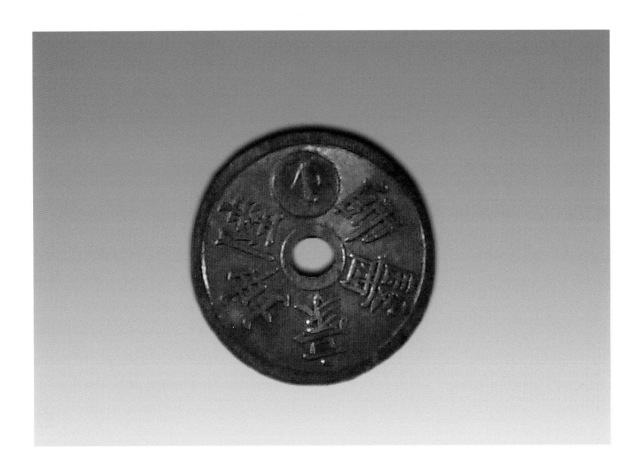

陆坤豪挂号牌

现代

铜质

直径 3 厘米，厚 0.1 厘米

Registration Tablet of Lu Kunhao

Modern Times

Copper

Diameter 3 cm/ Thickness 0.1 cm

圆形，为医事挂号牌。该藏用铜片制成，背面光滑，正面阳刻有"陆坤豪医师 4"字样，中心有圆孔。1955 年入藏。

中华医学会 / 上海中医药大学医史博物馆藏

The round tablet was made for medical registration. It was made of copper, with a smooth back and characters "Lu Kun Hao Yi Shi 4" meaning "Doctor Lu Kunhao 4" which was cut in relief on the surface. There is a hole in the middle. It was collected in 1955.

Preserved in Chinese Medical Association/ Museum of Chinese Medicine, Shanghai University of Traditional Chinese Medicine

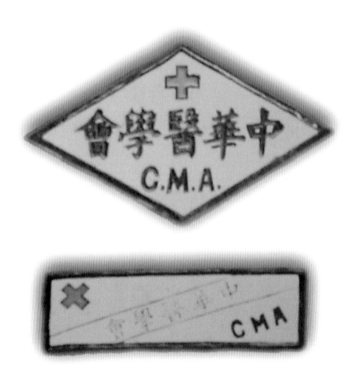

中华医学会徽章

现代

金属质地

菱形章：长 4.5 厘米，宽 2.5 厘米

方形章：长 4 厘米，宽 1.3 厘米

Badges of the Chinese Medical Association

Modern Times

Metal

The Rhombic One: Length 4.5 cm/ Width 2.5 cm

The Oblong One: Length 4 cm/ Width 1.3 cm

徽章。菱形、方形各一枚，表面有十字图案和
"中华医学会"及"C.M.A."字样。中华医学会
1915年成立于上海，主要从事医学著作的编辑翻
译、医学教育的研究、名词审定、医学标准的拟
定等学术活动及会员的福利工作等 。1961年入
藏。保存基本完好 。

中华医学会/上海中医药大学医史博物馆藏

There are two badges, a rhombic one and a oblong
one. The surfaces of both badges are decorated
with a cross pattern, characters reading "Zhong
Hua Yi Xue Hui" (Chinese Medical Association)
as well as English letters C.M.A. Chinese Medical
Association was established in Shanghai in 1915. Its
main duties were academic work such as compiling
and translating famous medical books, researching
medical education, examining and approving medical
terminology and standards, as well as maintaining
welfare of its members. The badges were collected
in 1961 and is well-preserved.

Preserved in Chinese Medical Association/Museum of
Chinese Medicine, Shanghai University of Traditional
Chinese Medicine

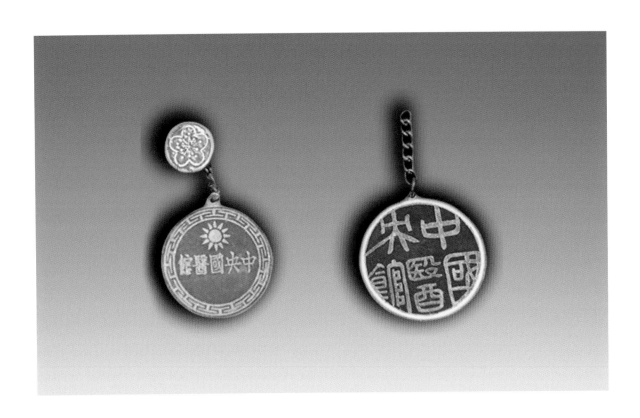

中央国医馆徽章

民国时期

金属质地

左：直径 2.6 厘米

右：直径 3 厘米

Badges of the Central State Hospital

Republican Period

Metal

The Left One: Diameter 2.6 cm

The Right One: Diameter 3 cm

徽章。1931 年国民政府为缓和中医界对其限制乃至消灭中医做法的抗争，在南京设立了中央国医馆，一些省、市、县也先后设立了分馆、支馆，对制订、整理学术标准大纲，统一病名和编审部分教材做了一些工作。

上海中医药博物馆藏

In 1931, the Central State Hospital was founded in Nanjing by the National Government in order to relax the tension between the Chinese medicine field and the National Government caused by its limitation and even forbidding towards Chinese medicine. Some provinces and cities successively established their branch hospitals and sub-hospitals. They worked for formulating and editing academic standard synopsis, unifying names of diseases, as well as checking and editing some of textbooks.

Preserved in Shanghai Museum of Traditional Chinese Medicine

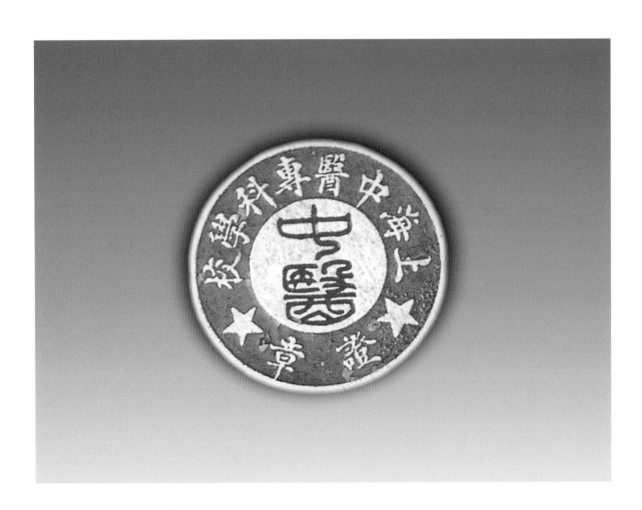

上海中医专科学校证章

近代

直径 2.75 厘米

Badge of Shanghai Traditional Chinese Medicine Specialized School

Modern Times

Diameter 2.75 cm

时逸人捐赠。时逸人〔1896—1966〕，江
苏省无锡人，现代医学家。与施今墨、张赞
臣、俞慎初等创办上海中医专科学校。编撰
上海中医专科学校第一届毕业纪念专刊，刊
于1940年《复兴中医》杂志第一卷第三期。

上海中医药博物馆藏

The badge was donated by Shi Yiren. Shi
Yiren (1896–1966), born in Wuxi City, Jiangsu
Province, was a modern medical scientist.
He co-founded Shanghai Traditional Chinese
Medicine Specialized School with Shi Jinmo,
Zhang Zanchen and Yu Shenchu and so on. He
compiled the first graduation commemorative
issue of Shanghai Chinese Medicine Specialized
School, which was published on *The Revival of
Traditional Chinese Medicine* (Issue 3, Vol. 1)
in 1940.

Preserved in Shanghai Museum of Traditional
Chinese Medicine

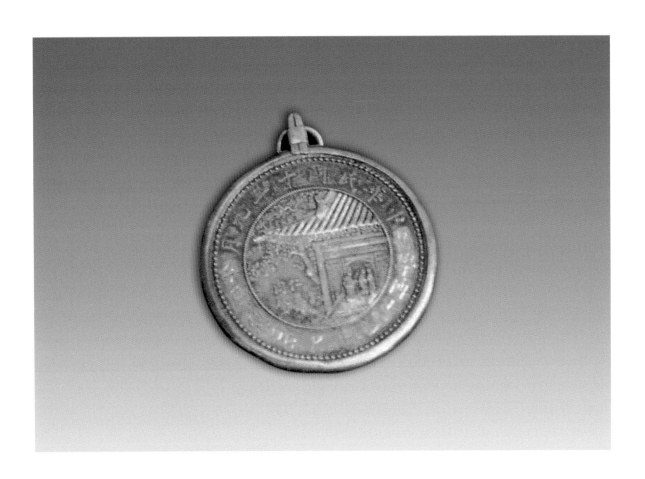

北京协和医院建院纪念章

民国时期

铜质

长 5 厘米，宽 4 厘米

Establishment Souvenir Badge of the Peking Union Medical College Hospital

Republican Period

Copper

Length 5 cm/ Width 4 cm

北京协和医院建成于 1921 年，由洛克菲勒
基金会创办。1942 年初，抗日战争北平沦陷
后停办。1948 年 5 月恢复。1951 年由中央
人民政府接管，隶属于中国医学科学院。

上海中医药博物馆藏

Peking Union Medical College Hospital was
established in 1921 by Rockefeller Foundation.
It was closed after the fall of Peking during the
Anti-Japanese War and was reopened in May
1948. In 1951, it was taken over by the Central
Government of PRC, and became affiliated to
Chinese Academy of Medical Sciences.
Preserved in Shanghai Museum of Traditional
Chinese Medicine

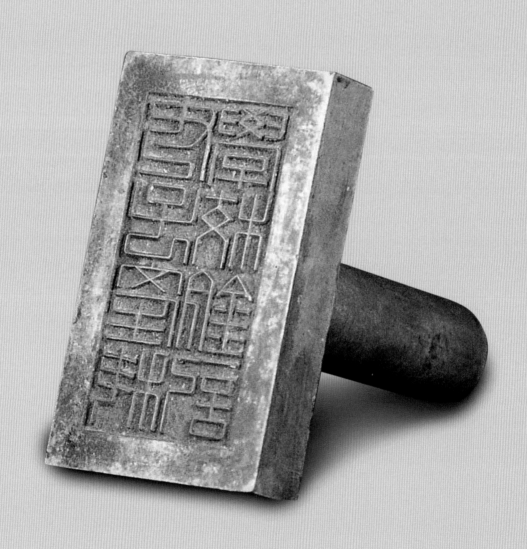

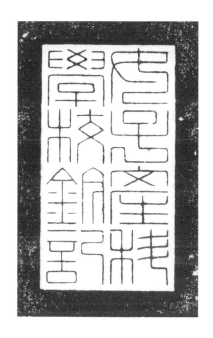

"女子产科学校" 印章

民国时期

铜质

长 8 厘米，宽 5.5 厘米，高 7.5 厘米

长方形，朱文，篆体。左图为其印蜕。民国元年（1912），汪惕予在上海创办女子产科学校。汪惕予（1869—1941），上海绩溪县人，光绪十九年（1893）学医，光绪二十三年（1897）在上海英租界中旺弄开设诊所。光绪三十年（1904）创办自新医科学校，并附设自新医院。

上海中医药博物馆藏

Seal of the Female Obstetrics School

Republican Period

Copper

Length 8 cm/ Width 5.5 cm/ Height 7.5 cm

The seal is oblong, with seal characters carved in relief on the surface. The picture on the right side is seal stamp. In the first reign year of the Republic of China (1912), Wang Tiyu founded the Female Obstetrics School in Shanghai. Wang Tiyu (1869–1941) was born in the Jixi County of Shanghai. He studied medicine in 1893 and opened a clinic in British concession of Shanghai in 1897. Then in 1904, he founded Zixin Medical School and Zixin Hospital as the affiliated institution.

Preserved in Shanghai Museum of Traditional Chinese Medicine

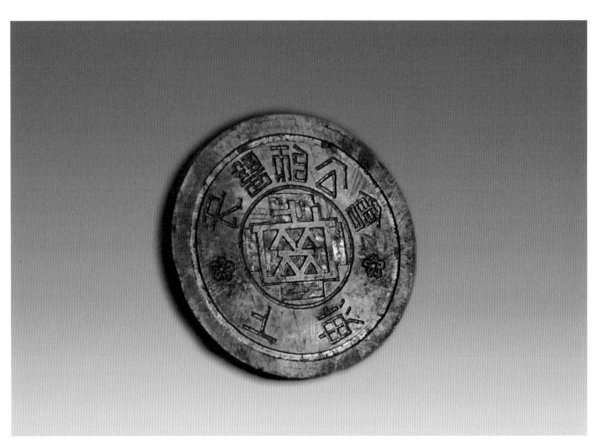

上海牙医师公会铜印

民国时期

铜质

直径 4.12 厘米，高 1.2 厘米

Copper Seal of Shanghai Dentist Association

Republican Period

Copper

Diameter 4.12 cm/ Height 1.2 cm

圆形，公章。由前上海市牙医师公会捐赠，

该会详情待考。1959 年入藏。基本完好，印

面有污迹。

中华医学会／上海中医药大学医史博物馆藏

It is a round official seal donated by the former
Shanghai Dentist Association. The details of
this association remain to be verified. It was
collected in 1959. It is basically well-preserved.
There is some smudge on it.

Preserved in Chinese Medical Association/
Museum of Chinese Medicine, Shanghai
University of Traditional Chinese Medicine

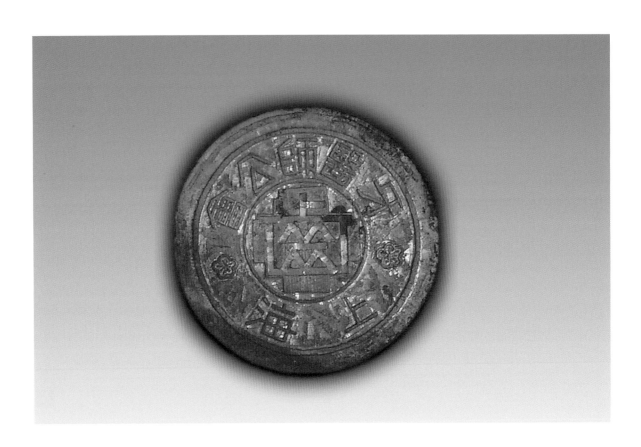

上海牙医师公会铜印

民国时期

铜质

直径 4.12 厘米，残高 0.37 厘米

Copper Seal of Shanghai Dental Association

Republican Period

Copper

Diameter 4.12 cm/ Residual Height 0.37 cm

圆形，公章。由前上海市牙医师公会捐赠，该会详情待考。1959 年入藏。基本完好，印面有污迹，印钮残缺。

中华医学会 / 上海中医药大学医史博物馆藏

It is a round official seal donated by the former Shanghai Dentist Association. The details of this association remain to be verified. It was collected in 1959. It is basically well-preserved. There is some smudge on it.

Preserved in Chinese Medical Association/ Museum of Chinese Medicine, Shanghai University of Traditional Chinese Medicine

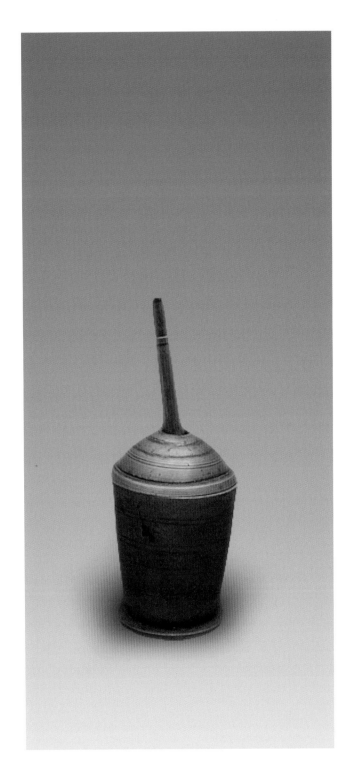

杵臼

民国时期

铜质

口径 10 厘米，高 11.5 厘米，盖高 4.5 厘米

Mortar with Pestle

Republican Period

Copper

Mouth Diameter 10 cm/ Height 11.5 cm/

Height of Lid 4.5 cm

平口，深腹，呈钵形，饼形足，穹隆形盖，盖顶有圆孔，用于杵穿过，腹部有四条刻线纹，足底饰铭文一圈。整器为黄铜色。保存完好。由民间征集。

　　成都中医药大学中医药传统文化博物馆藏

The mortar is like an alms bowl, with a flat mouth, a deep belly, a pie-shaped bottom, and an archivolt lid. There is a hole on the top of the lid for the pestle passing through it. There are four-cord designs on the belly and a ring of inscriptions on the bottom. It is of the colour of brass. It was collected from the folk and is well preserved now.

Preserved in Museum of Traditional Chinese Medicine Culture, Chengdu University of Traditional Chinese Medicine

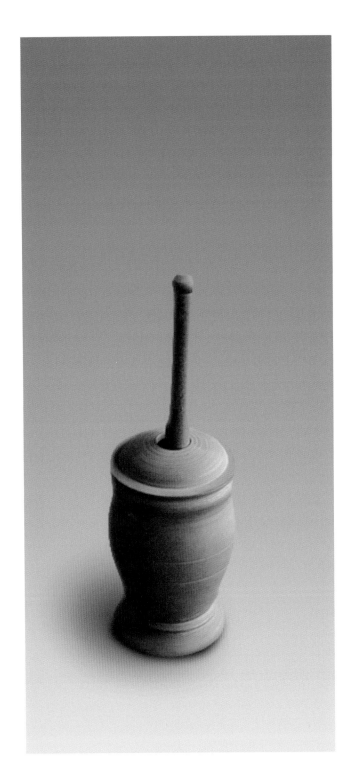

臼

民国时期

铜质

口径 9 厘米，底径 9 厘米，高 14 厘米，杵
长 14 厘米

Mortar

Republican Period

Copper

Mouth Diameter 9 cm/ Bottom Diameter 9 cm/
Height 14 cm/ Length of the Pestle 14 cm

圆口，腹稍鼓，饼形足，腹上有旋纹，盖中有孔，可使杵穿过，局部残。由民间征集。

成都中医药大学中医药传统文化博物馆藏

The mortar has a round mouth, a slightly bulged belly, and a pie-shaped bottom. There are spiral patterns around the belly. There is a hole in the middle of the lid for the pestle passing through it. Some parts of the mortar are incomplete. It was collected from the folk.

Preserved in Museum of Traditional Chinese Medicine Culture, Chengdu University of Traditional Chinese Medicine

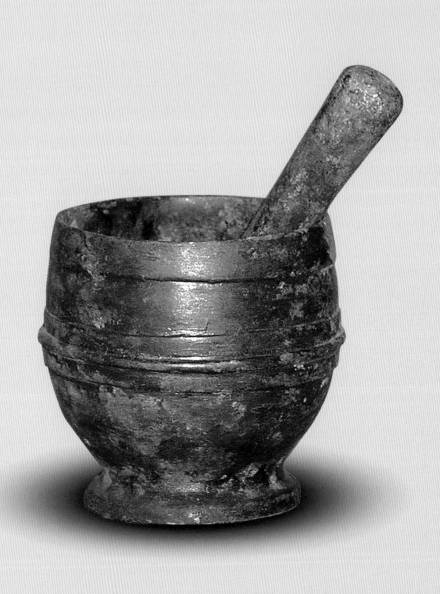

铜药臼

近代

铜质

口径 6 厘米，底径 4.8 厘米，通高 6 厘米，重 400 克

直口，鼓腹，平底，中腹有凸棱，带一杵。捣药器具。完整无损。

陕西医史博物馆藏

Copper Medicinal Mortar

Modern

Copper

Mouth Diameter 6 cm/ Bottom Diameter 4.8 cm/ Height 6 cm/ Weight 400 g

The mortar has a straight mouth, a bulged belly, and a flat bottom. There is a ring of bulged bridge around the belly. It also has a pestle. The mortar is used for smashing Chinese medicine. It is well-preserved now.

Preserved in Shaanxi Museum of Medical History

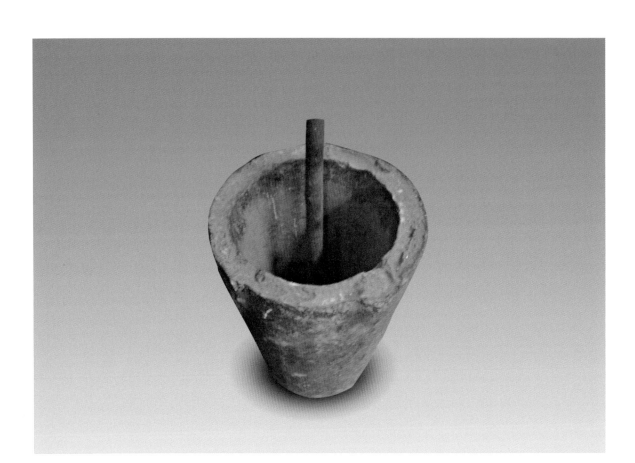

药臼

民国时期

铁质

直径 41 厘米，高 51 厘米

Medicinal Mortar

Republican Period

Iron

Diameter 41 cm/ Height 51 cm

形体较大，平口，深腹内收，配有一长形铁杆，用于舂制较大较硬的药材。由民间征集。

　　成都中医药大学中医药传统文化博物馆藏

The mortar is larger than normal size, with a flat mouth, a deep belly and a narrow bottom. It is equipped with a long gavelock for pestling larger and harder medicinal materials. It was collected from the folk.

Preserved in Museum of Traditional Chinese Medicine Culture, Chengdu University of Traditional Chinese Medicine

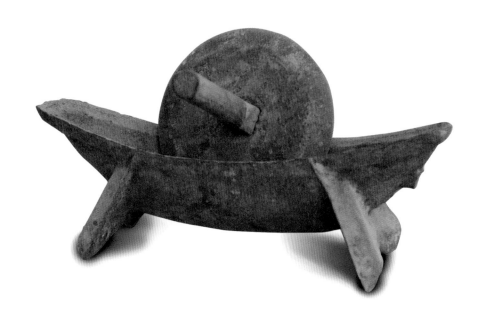

小铁药碾

现代

铁质

通长 31.5 厘米，底长 23 厘米，高 10.5 厘米，重 4700 克

船形有一槽，八字足，带一碾饼。药具。完整无损。

陕西医史博物馆藏

Small Iron Medicinal Crusher

Modern Times

Iron

Full-Length 31.5 cm/ Length of the Bottom 23 cm/ Height 10.5 cm/ Weight 4,700 g

The medicinal crusher is cymbiform with a groove. It also has splayed feet and a cake-shaped grind. It is a well-preserved medicinal instrument.

Preserved in Shaanxi Museum of Medical History

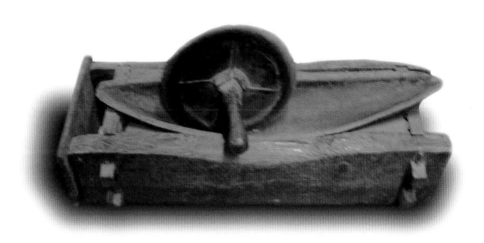

药碾船

民国时期

铁质

长 83 厘米，宽 35 厘米，高 25 厘米

带木质碾座，碾轮为铁质，配木手柄。保存完好。由民间征集。

成都中医药大学中医药传统文化博物馆藏

Ship-like Medicinal Crusher

Republican Period

Iron

Length 83 cm/ Width 35 cm/ Height 25 cm

It has a wooden grind-bottom, an iron runner wheel, and a wooden hand shank. It is well-preserved and was collected from the folk.

Preserved in Museum of Traditional Chinese Medicine Culture, Chengdu University of Traditional Chinese Medicine

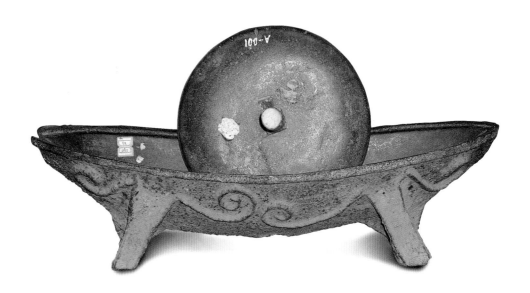

铁碾槽

革命战争时期

铁质

长 70 厘米，宽 20 厘米，通高 15.5 厘米，重 2000 克

呈船形，槽身有波浪纹两足。制药工具。有残。陕西省延安市征集。

陕西医史博物馆藏

Iron Mill Groove

The Period of the Revolutionary War

Iron

Length 70 cm/ Width 20 cm/ Height 15.5 cm/ Weight 2,000 g

The two-feet groove is cymbiform decorated with ripple patterns under its body. It is a pharmacy instrument, and some parts of it are damaged. It was collected from Yan'an City, Shaanxi Province.

Preserved in Shaanxi Museum of Medical History

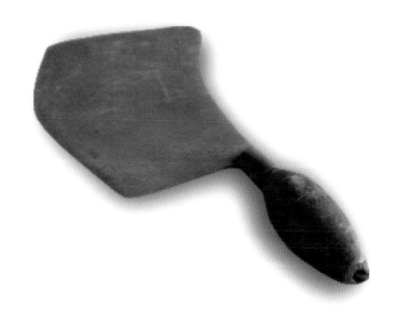

刀

民国时期

铁质

长 25 厘米

该藏为近代药房切药用具。由民间征集。

成都中医药大学中医药传统文化博物馆藏

Knife

Republican Period

Iron

Length 25 cm

The knife was used to cut medicine in Chinese medicine dispensary during the Modern Times. It was collected from the folk.

Preserved in Museum of Traditional Chinese Medicine Culture, Chengdu University of Traditional Chinese Medicine

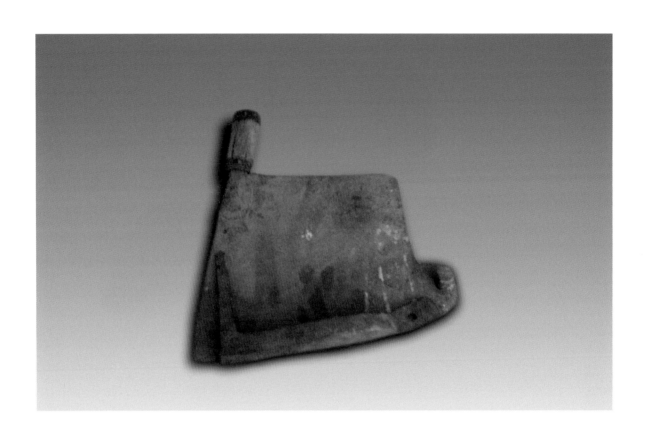

铁药刀

民国时期

铁质

长 29.5 厘米，宽 26 厘米，重 1500 克

Iron Medicinal Knife

Republican Period

Iron

Length 29.5 cm/ Width 26 cm/ Weight 1,500 g

刀状，带一圆木把及一铁钩。制药工具。完
整无损。陕西省延安市征集。

陕西医史博物馆藏

It is knife-shaped, with a round wooden
handle and an iron cleek. It is a well preserved
pharmaceutical instrument. It was collected
from Yan'an City, Shaanxi Province.

Preserved in Shaanxi Museum of Medical History

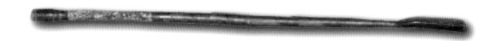

铜药匙

民国时期

铜质

长 14 厘米，重 1 克

头为铲状，柄为长圆形。完整无损。

陕西医史博物馆藏

Copper Medicinal Spoon

Republican Period

Copper

Length 14 cm/ Weight 1 g

The spoon has a shovel-shaped head, and a long and cylindrical handle. It is well-preserved.

Preserved in Shaanxi Museum of Medical History

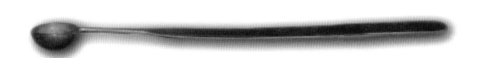

铜药勺

民国时期

铜质

长 21.2 厘米，宽 2.2 厘米，重 50 克

勺头小深，勺柄前端细圆，后柄呈扁平状。药具。完整无损。内蒙古征集。

陕西医史博物馆藏

Copper Medicinal Ladle

Republican Period

Copper

Length 21.2 cm/ Width 2.2 cm/ Weight 50 g

The head of the ladle is small and deep. The front-end of the handle is a thin cylinder. The after-end of the handle is tabular. It is a well preserved pharmaceutical instrument. It was collected from the Inner Mongolia.

Preserved in Shaanxi Museum of Medical History

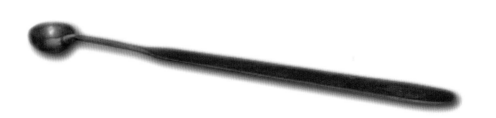

铜药勺

民国时期

铜质

长 21.2 厘米，宽 2.2 厘米，重 50 克

勺头小深，勺柄前端细圆，后柄呈扁平状。 药具。完整无损。内蒙古征集。

陕西医史博物馆藏

Copper Medicinal Ladle

Republican Period

Copper

Length 21.2 cm/ Width 2.2 cm/ Weight 50 g

The head of the ladle is small and deep. The front-end of the handle is a thin cylinder. The after-end of the handle is tabular. It is a well preserved pharmaceutical instrument. It was collected from the Inner Mongolia.

Preserved in Shaanxi Museum of Medical History

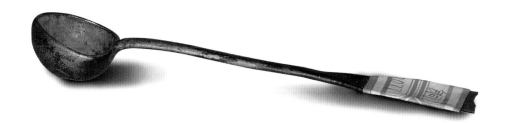

铜药勺

民国时期

铜质

长 14 厘米，宽 3 厘米，重 50 克

勺头小深，勺柄前端细圆，后柄呈扁平状。药具。有残。

陕西医史博物馆藏

Copper Medicinal Ladle

Republican Period

Copper

Length 14 cm/ Width 3 cm/ Weight 50 g

The head of the ladle is small and deep. The front-end of the handle is a thin cylinder. The after-end of the handle is tabular. It is a pharmaceutical instrument, and some parts of it are damaged.

Preserved in Shaanxi Museum of Medical History

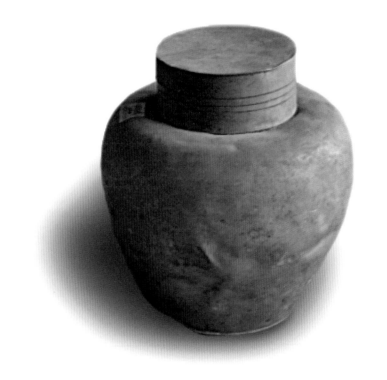

药罐

民国时期

锡质

腹径 18.5 厘米，高 17 厘米

直口，鼓肩，腹内收，平底，有盖与口相扣。由民间征集。

成都中医药大学中医药传统文化博物馆藏

Gallipot

Republican Period

Tin

Belly Mouth Diameter 18.5 cm/ Height 17 cm

The gallipot has a straight mouth, a drum-like shoulder, an oblique belly and a flat bottom. There is also a lid which can button with the mouth. It was collected from the folk.

Preserved in Museum of Traditional Chinese Medicine Culture, Chengdu University of Traditional Chinese Medicine

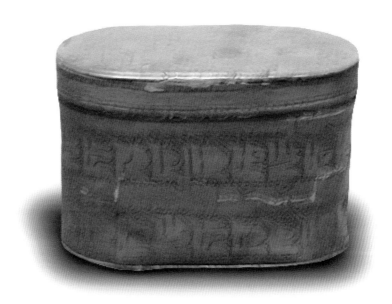

药盒

民国时期

铜质

长 8 厘米，宽 4.5 厘米，高 6 厘米

由民间征集。

成都中医药大学中医药传统文化博物馆藏

Medicine Box

Republican Period

Copper

Length 8 cm/ Width 4.5 cm/ Height 6 cm

The medicine box was collected from the folk.

Preserved in Museum of Traditional Chinese Medicine Culture, Chengdu University of Traditional Chinese Medicine

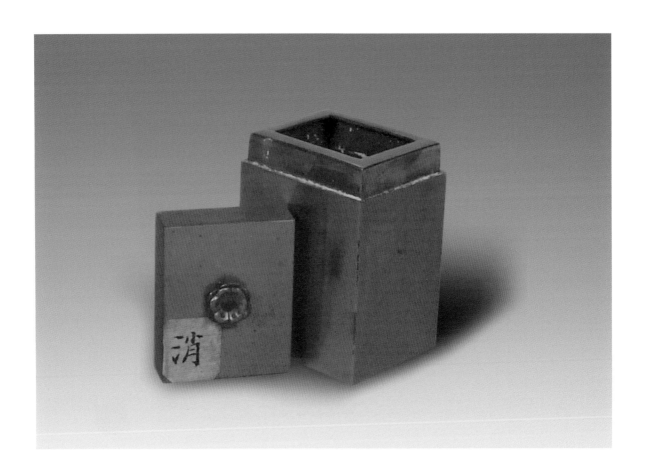

药盒

民国时期

合金

长 3.1 厘米，宽 3.7 厘米，高 5.3 厘米

Medicine Box

Republican Period

Alloy

Length 3.1 cm/ Width 3.7 cm/ Height 5.3 cm

方形，用于盛药。该藏为该馆自购的民国时
期红木药箱中的盛药器皿之一，该药箱曾为
南翔张志方中医室所用，是张氏庚申年购置
于姑苏之品。该藏合金铸造，工艺精湛，造
型优美，盒盖花瓣式小钮，贴有"消"字标记。
1959 年入藏。保存基本完好。

中华医学会 / 上海中医药大学医史博物馆藏

The square box was used for storing medicine
and was one of the receptacles for medicine in
the mahogany medicine chest in the Republican
Period which the museum bought itself. This
chest was once used by Doctor Zhang Zhifang's
TCM clinic in Nanxiang. It was bought by him
when he was in Suzhou City in 1920. The box is
alloy casting by using sophisticated technology,
and has an aesthetic outline. There is a petal-
like knob and a label bearing a character " 消 "
(Xiao) on the lid. It was collected in 1959 and is
still in good condition.

Preserved in Chinese Medical Association/
Museum of Chinese Medicine, Shanghai
University of Traditional Chinese Medicine

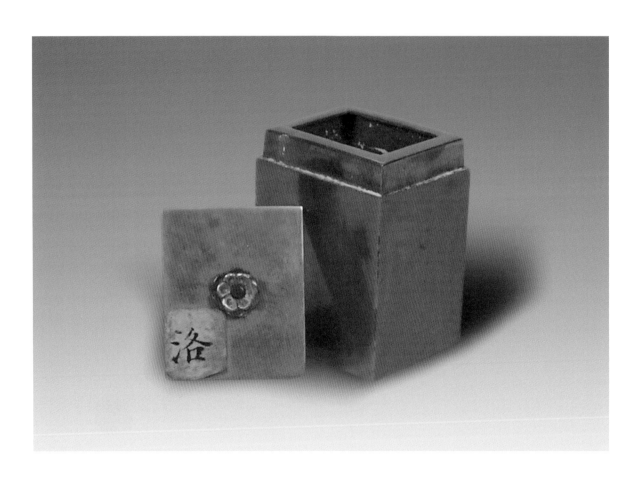

药盒

民国时期

合金

长 3.1 厘米，宽 3.7 厘米，高 5.3 厘米

Medicine Box

Republican Period

Alloy

Length 3.1 cm/ Width 3.7 cm/ Height 5.3 cm

方形，用于盛药。该藏为该馆自购的民国时期红木药箱中的盛药器皿之一，该药箱曾为南翔张志方中医室所用，是张氏庚申年购置于姑苏之品。该藏合金铸造，工艺精湛，造型优美，盒盖花瓣式小钮，贴有"洛"字标记。1959 年入藏。保存基本完好。

中华医学会 / 上海中医药大学医史博物馆藏

The square box was used for storing medicine and was one of the receptacles for medicine in the mahogany medicine chest in the Republican Period which the museum bought itself. This chest was once used by Doctor Zhang Zhifang's TCM clinic in Nanxiang. It was bought by him when he was in Suzhou City in 1920. The box is alloy casting by using sophisticated technology, and has an aesthetic outline. There is a petal-like knob and a label bearing a character " 洛 " (Luo) on the lid. It was collected in 1959 and is still in good condition.

Preserved in Chinese Medical Association/ Museum of Chinese Medicine, Shanghai University of Traditional Chinese Medicine

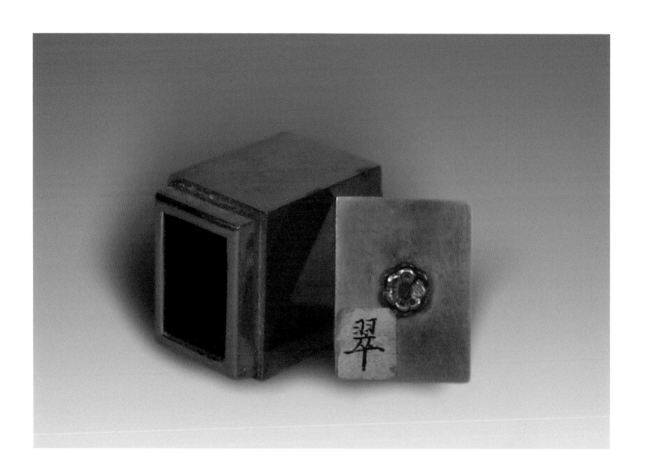

药盒

民国时期

合金

长 3.1 厘米，宽 3.7 厘米，高 5.3 厘米

Medicine Box

Republican Period

Alloy

Length 3.1 cm/ Width 3.7 cm/ Height 5.3 cm

方形，用于盛药。该藏为该馆自购的民国红
木药箱中的盛药器皿之一，该药箱曾为南翔
张志方中医室所用，是张氏庚申年购置于姑
苏之品。该藏工艺精湛，造型优美，盒盖花
瓣式小钮，贴有"翠"字标记。1959 年入藏。
保存基本完好。

中华医学会 / 上海中医药大学医史博物馆藏

The square box was used for storing medicine
and was one of the receptacles for medicine in
the mahogany medicine chest in the Republican
Period which the museum bought itself. This
chest was once used by Doctor Zhang Zhifang's
TCM clinic in Nanxiang. It was bought by him
when he was in Suzhou City in 1920. The box is
alloy casting by using sophisticated technology,
and has an aesthetic outline. There is a petal-
like knob and a label bearing a character " 翠 "
(Cui) on the lid. It was collected in 1959 and is
still in good condition.
Preserved in Chinese Medical Association/
Museum of Chinese Medicine, Shanghai
University of Traditional Chinese Medicine

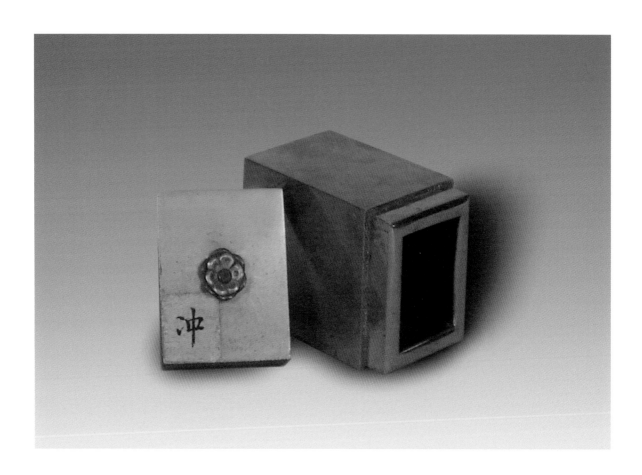

药盒

民国时期

合金

长 3.1 厘米，宽 3.7 厘米，高 5.3 厘米

Medicine Box

Republican Period

Alloy

Length 3.1 cm/ Width 3.7 cm/ Height 5.3 cm

方形，用于盛药。该藏为该馆自购的民国时
期红木药箱中的盛药器皿之一，该药箱曾为
南翔张志方中医室所用，是张氏庚申年购置
于姑苏之品。该藏合金铸造，工艺精湛，造
型优美，盒盖花瓣式小钮，贴有"冲"字标记。
1959 年入藏。保存基本完好。

中华医学会 / 上海中医药大学医史博物馆藏

The square box was used for storing medicine
and was one of the receptacles for medicine
in the mahogany medicine chest in the
Republican Period which the museum bought
itself. This chest was once used by Doctor
Zhang Zhifang's TCM clinic in Nanxiang. It
was bought by him when he was in Suzhou
City in 1920. The box is alloy casting by using
sophisticated technology, and has an aesthetic
outline. There is a petal-like knob and a label
bearing a character " 冲 " (Chong) on the lid.
It was collected in 1959 and is still in good
condition.
Preserved in Chinese Medical Association/
Museum of Chinese Medicine, Shanghai
University of Traditional Chinese Medicine

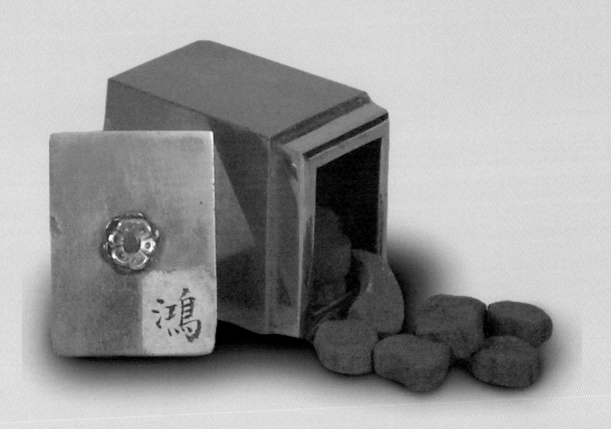

药盒

民国时期

合金

长 3.1 厘米，宽 3.7 厘米，高 5.3 厘米

Medicine Box

Republican Period

Alloy

Length 3.1 cm/ Width 3.7 cm/ Height 5.3 cm

方形，用于盛药。该藏为该馆自购的民国时期红木药箱中的盛药器皿之一，该药箱曾为南翔张志方中医室所用，是张氏庚申年购置于姑苏之品。该藏合金铸造，工艺精湛，造型优美，盒盖花瓣式小钮，贴有"鸿"字标记。1959 年入藏。保存基本完好。

中华医学会 / 上海中医药大学医史博物馆藏

The square box was used for storing medicine and was one of the receptacles for medicine in the mahogany medicine chest in the Republican Period which the museum bought itself. This chest was once used by Doctor Zhang Zhifang's TCM clinic in Nanxiang. It was bought by him when he was in Suzhou City in 1920. The box is alloy casting by using sophisticated technology, and has an aesthetic outline. There is a petal-like knob and a label bearing a character " 鸿 " (Hong) on the lid. It was collected in 1959 and is still in good condition.

Preserved in Chinese Medical Association/ Museum of Chinese Medicine, Shanghai University of Traditional Chinese Medicine

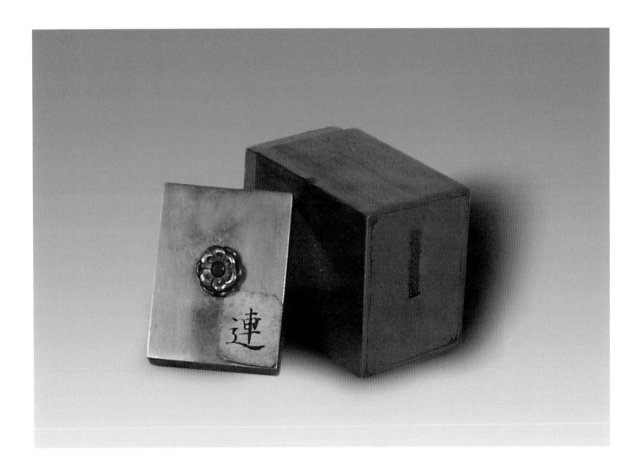

药盒

民国时期

合金

长 3.1 厘米，宽 3.7 厘米，高 5.3 厘米

Medicine Box

Republican Period

Alloy

Length 3.1 cm/ Width 3.7 cm/ Height 5.3 cm

方形，用于盛药。该藏为该馆自购的民国时期红木药箱中的盛药器皿之一，该药箱曾为南翔张志方中医室所用，是张氏庚申年购置于姑苏之品。该藏工艺精湛，造型优美，盒盖花瓣式小钮，贴有"连"字标记。1959年入藏。保存基本完好。

中华医学会/上海中医药大学医史博物馆藏

The square box was used for storing medicine and was one of the receptacles for medicine in the mahogany medicine chest in the Republican Period which the museum bought itself. This chest was once used by Doctor Zhang Zhifang's TCM clinic in Nanxiang. It was bought by him when he was in Suzhou City in 1920. The box is alloy casting by using sophisticated technology, and has an aesthetic outline. There is a petal-like knob and a label bearing a character "连" (Lian) on the lid. It was collected in 1959 and is still in good condition.

Preserved in Chinese Medical Association/ Museum of Chinese Medicine, Shanghai University of Traditional Chinese Medicine

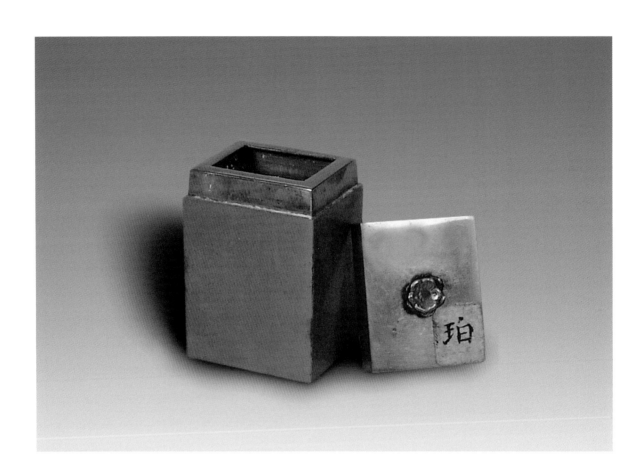

药盒

民国时期

合金

长 3.1 厘米，宽 3.7 厘米，高 5.3 厘米

Medicine Box

Republican Period

Alloy

Length 3.1 cm/ Width 3.7 cm/ Height 5.3 cm

方形，用于盛药。该藏为该馆自购的民国时
期红木药箱中的盛药器皿之一，该药箱曾为
南翔张志方中医室所用，是张氏庚申年购置
于姑苏之品。该藏合金铸造，工艺精湛，造
型优美，盒盖花瓣式小钮，贴有"珀"字标记。
1959 年入藏。保存基本完好。

中华医学会 / 上海中医药大学医史博物馆藏

The square box was used for storing medicine
and was one of the receptacles for medicine in
the mahogany medicine chest in the Republican
Period which the museum bought itself. This
chest was once used by Doctor Zhang Zhifang's
TCM clinic in Nanxiang. It was bought by him
when he was in Suzhou City in 1920. The box is
alloy casting by using sophisticated technology,
and has an aesthetic outline. There is a petal-
like knob and a label bearing a character " 珀 "
(Po) on the lid. It was collected in 1959 and is
still in good condition.

Preserved in Chinese Medical Association/
Museum of Chinese Medicine, Shanghai
University of Traditional Chinese Medicine

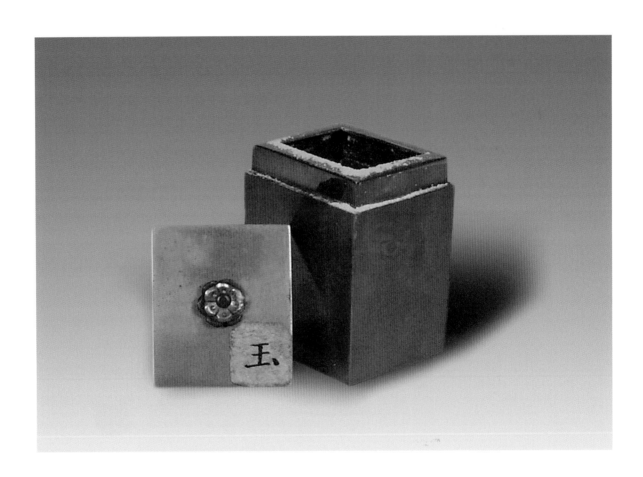

药盒

民国时期

合金

长 3.1 厘米，宽 3.7 厘米，高 5.3 厘米

Medicine Box

Republican Period

Alloy

Length 3.1 cm/ Width 3.7 cm/ Height 5.3 cm

方形，用于盛药。该藏为该馆自购的民国红木药箱中的盛药器皿之一，该药箱曾为南翔张志方中医室所用，是张氏庚申年购置于姑苏之品。该藏合金铸造，工艺精湛，造型优美，盒盖花瓣式小钮，贴有"玉"字标记。1959年入藏。保存基本完好。

中华医学会/上海中医药大学医史博物馆藏

The square box was used for storing medicine and was one of the receptacles for medicine in the mahogany medicine chest in the Republican Period which the museum bought itself. This chest was once used by Doctor Zhang Zhifang's TCM clinic in Nanxiang. It wast by him when he was in Suzhou City in 1920. The box is alloy casting by using sophisticated technology, and has an aesthetic outline. There is a petal-like knob and a label bearing a character "玉" (Yu) on the lid. It was collected in 1959 and is still in good condition.

Preserved in Chinese Medical Association/ Museum of Chinese Medicine, Shanghai University of Traditional Chinese Medicine

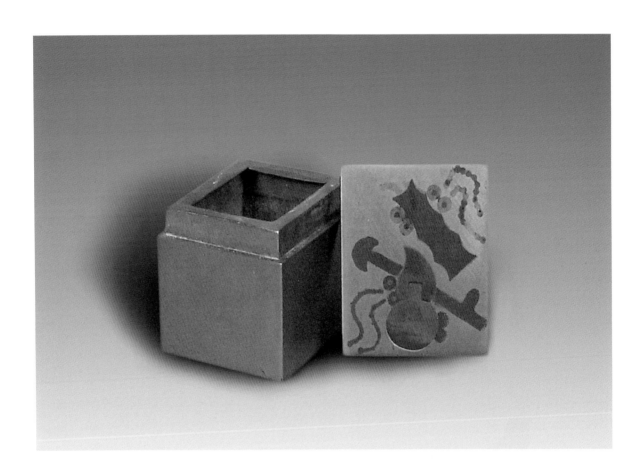

药盒

民国时期

合金

长 3.8 厘米，宽 3.3 厘米，高 3.3 厘米

Medicine Box

Republican Period

Alloy

Length 3.8 cm/ Width 3.3 cm/ Height 3.3 cm

方形，用于盛药。该藏为该馆自购的民国时期红木药箱中的盛药器皿之一，该药箱曾为南翔张志方中医室所用，是张氏庚申年购置于姑苏之品。该藏工艺精湛，造型优美，盒盖镶嵌纹饰及掀开式暗拉手。1959 年入藏。保存基本完好。

中华医学会 / 上海中医药大学医史博物馆藏

The square kit was used for storing medicine and was one of the receptacles for medicine in the mahogany medicine chest purchase by the museum. The chest was once used in Doctor Zhang Zhifang's TCM clinic in Nanxiang and It was bought by Zhang in Gusu (now Suzhou) in 1920. In refined form and intricately worked design, the kit was engraved with patterns on the lid and has a hidden handle which needs to be lifted before holding. It was collected in 1959 and is still in good condition.

Preserved in Chinese Medical Association/ Museum of Chinese Medicine, Shanghai University of Traditional Chinese Medicine

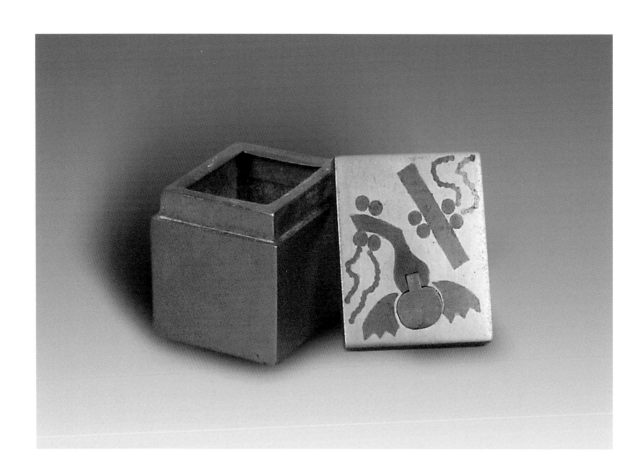

药盒

民国时期

合金

长 3.8 厘米，宽 3.3 厘米，高 3.3 厘米

Medicine Box

Republican Period

Alloy

Length 3.8 cm/ Width 3.3 cm/ Height 3.3 cm

方形，用于盛药。该藏为该馆自购的民国时期红木药箱中的盛药器皿之一，该药箱曾为南翔张志方中医室所用，是张氏庚申年置于姑苏之品。该藏工艺精湛，造型优美，盒盖镶嵌纹饰及掀开式暗拉手。1959年入藏。保存基本完好。

中华医学会/上海中医药大学医史博物馆藏

The square kit was used for storing medicine and was one of the receptacles for medicine in the mahogany medicine chest purchase by the museum. The chest was once used in Doctor Zhang Zhifang's TCM clinic in Nanxiang and It was bought by Zhang in Gusu (now Suzhou) in 1920. In refined form and intricately worked design, the kit was engraved with patterns on the lid and has a hidden handle which needs to be lifted before holding. It was collected in 1959 and is still in good condition.

Preserved in Chinese Medical Association/ Museum of Chinese Medicine, Shanghai University of Traditional Chinese Medicine

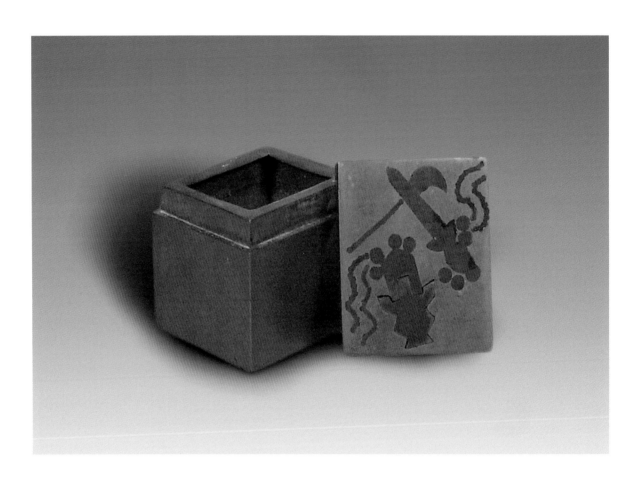

药盒

民国时期

合金

长 3.8 厘米，宽 3.3 厘米，高 3.3 厘米

Medicine Box

Republican Period

Alloy

Length 3.8 cm/ Width 3.3 cm/ Height 3.3 cm

方形，用于盛药。该藏为该馆自购的民国时期红木药箱中的盛药器皿之一，该药箱曾为南翔张志方中医室所用，是张氏庚申年购置于姑苏之品。该藏工艺精湛，造型优美，盒盖镶嵌纹饰及掀开式暗拉手。1959 年入藏。保存基本完好。

中华医学会 / 上海中医药大学医史博物馆藏

The square kit was used for storing medicine and was one of the receptacles for medicine in the mahogany medicine chest purchase by the museum. The chest was once used in Doctor Zhang Zhifang's TCM clinic in Nanxiang and It was bought by Zhang in Gusu (now Suzhou) in 1920. In refined form and intricately worked design, the kit was engraved with patterns on the lid and has a hidden handle which needs to be lifted before holding. It was collected in 1959 and is still in good condition.

Preserved in Chinese Medical Association/ Museum of Chinese Medicine, Shanghai University of Traditional Chinese Medicine

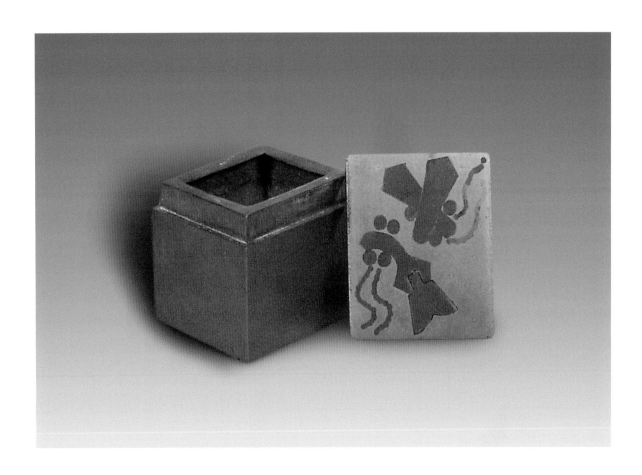

药盒

民国时期

合金

长 3.8 厘米，宽 3.3 厘米，高 3.3 厘米

Medicine Box

Republican Period

Alloy

Length 3.8 cm/ Width 3.3 cm/ Height 3.3 cm

方形，用于盛药。该藏为该馆自购的民国时期红木药箱中的盛药器皿之一，该药箱曾为南翔张志方中医室所用，是张氏庚申年购置于姑苏之品。该藏工艺精湛，造型优美，盒盖镶嵌纹饰及掀开式暗拉手。1959 年入藏。保存基本完好。

中华医学会 / 上海中医药大学医史博物馆藏

The square kit was used for storing medicine and was one of the receptacles for medicine in the mahogany medicine chest purchase by the museum. The chest was once used in Doctor Zhang Zhifang's TCM clinic in Nanxiang and It was bought by Zhang in Gusu (now Suzhou) in 1920. In refined form and intricately worked design, the kit was engraved with patterns on the lid and has a hidden handle which needs to be lifted before holding. It was collected in 1959 and is still in good condition.

Preserved in Chinese Medical Association/ Museum of Chinese Medicine, Shanghai University of Traditional Chinese Medicine

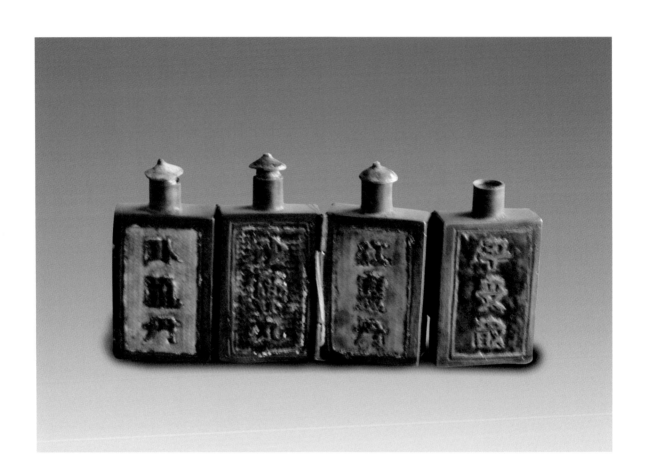

药瓶

现代

锡质

长 8.5 厘米，宽 3 厘米

Medicine Bottles

Modern Times

Tin

Length 8.5 cm/ Width 3 cm

该藏由四个独立的方形药瓶相连而成，用于

存放粉状药物。

　　成都中医药大学中医药传统文化博物馆藏

Four independent medicine bottles are joined
one to another as a whole with hinges for
storing medicine powder.

Preserved in Museum of Traditional Chinese
Medicine Culture, Chengdu University of Traditional
Chinese Medicine

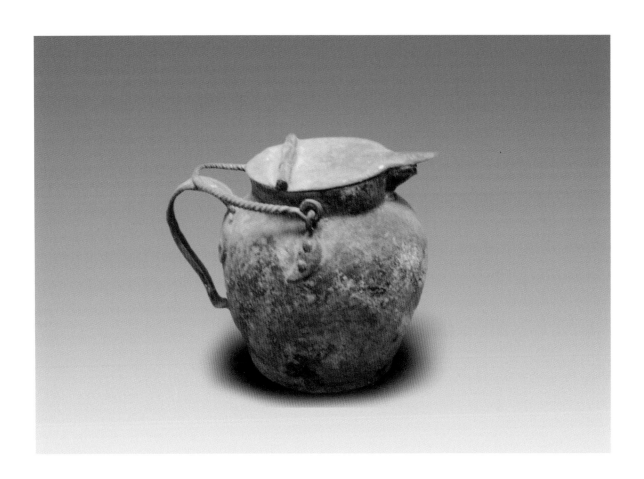

煎药罐

民国时期

锡质

高 21 厘米

The Pot for Decocting Herbal Medicine

Republican Period

Tin

Height 21 cm

直口，鼓腹，平底，肩部有两个对称的环形耳，耳上系有饰纹状的提梁，腹部有一把，口部有流，盖呈鸭嘴形，一端固定在口部。保存完好。由民间征集。

成都中医药大学中医药传统文化博物馆藏

The pot has a straight mouth, a swelling belly, a flat bottom, two symmetric ring-like ears on shoulders, a patterned hoop handle attached to ears, a handle on the belly, a spout in the mouth, and a lid in form of the duck's bill, with one end fixed in the mouth. It was collected from the folk and is still in good condition.

Preserved in Museum of Traditional Chinese Medicine Culture, Chengdu University of Traditional Chinese Medicine

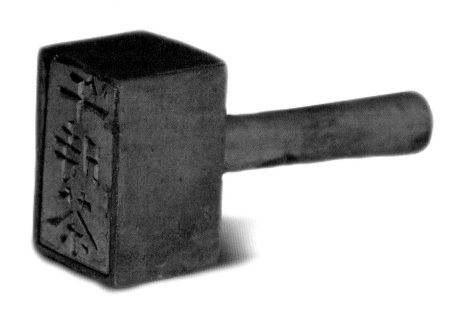

"午时茶" 模具

近代

铜质

模腔：长 5.2 厘米，宽 3.5 厘米，深 2.8 厘米

模托：长 11 厘米

"Wu Shi Cha" (Herbal Tea) Mould

Modern Times

Copper

Mould Cavity: Length 5.2 cm/ Width 3.5 cm/ Depth 2.8 cm

Mould Handle: Length 11 cm

该藏为药坊制作药砖的模具，刻有"午时
茶"字样。制出的药砖尺寸为 4.6 厘米×3 厘
米×2.8 厘米。

北京中医药大学中医药博物馆藏

Engraved with three characters reading "Wu
Shi Sha" (herbal tea), the mould is used in
pharmacy to make medicine bricks in size of
4.6 cm×3 cm×2.8 cm.

Preserved in Museum of Chinese Medicine,
Beijing University of Chinese Medicine

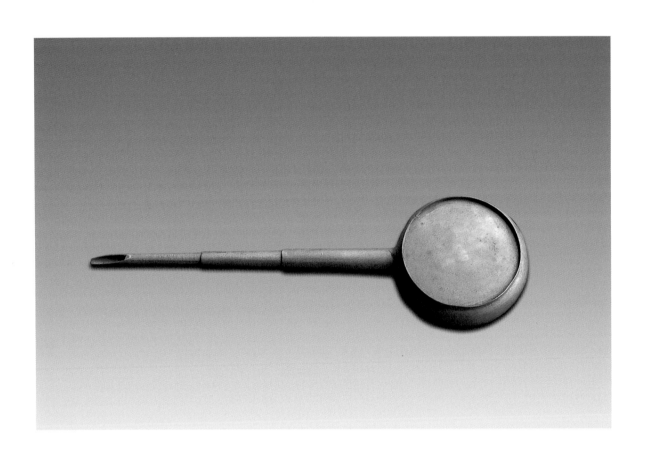

鼻箔管

近代

铜质

直径 4 厘米，长 13 厘米

Nasal Tube Covered with Foil

Mordern Times

Copper

Diameter 4 cm/ Length 13 cm

用于咽喉部疾病吹药。体作圆鼓形，铜管多节。使用时，挤压圆鼓，可使药粉吹至病患处。

江苏省中医药博物馆藏

The nasal tube was used to blow the medicine to the pharynx or larynx. It is an instrument with a drum-like belly and a multi-section copper handle. When pressing the drum-like belly, the medicine powder can be blown to the affected part.

Preserved in Jiangsu Museum of Traditional Chinese Medicine

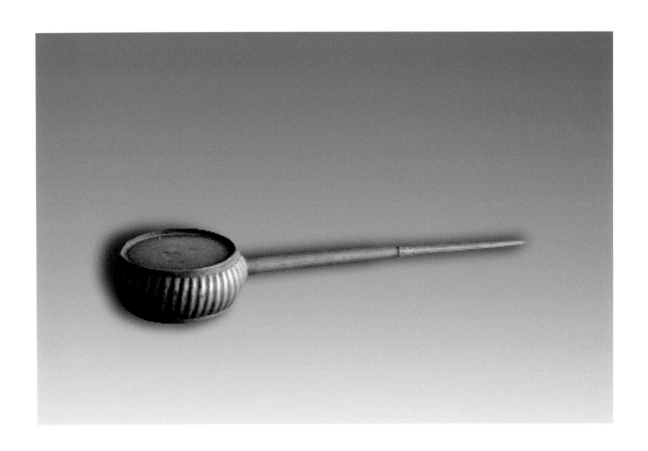

药鼓

民国时期

铜质

直径 4.5 厘米，长 16 厘米

Drum-like Medical Instrument

Republican Period

Copper

Diameter 4.5 cm/ Length 16 cm

吹药用具。体作圆鼓形，铜管多节。使用时，挤压圆鼓，可使药粉吹至病患处。由民间征集。

　　成都中医药大学中医药传统文化博物馆藏

The drum-like medical instrument was used for applying medicine. It is an instrument with a drum-like belly and a multi-section copper handle. When pressing the drum-like belly, the medicine powder can be blown to the affected part. It was collected from the folk.

Preserved in Museum of Traditional Chinese Medicine Culture, Chengdu University of Traditional Chinese Medicine

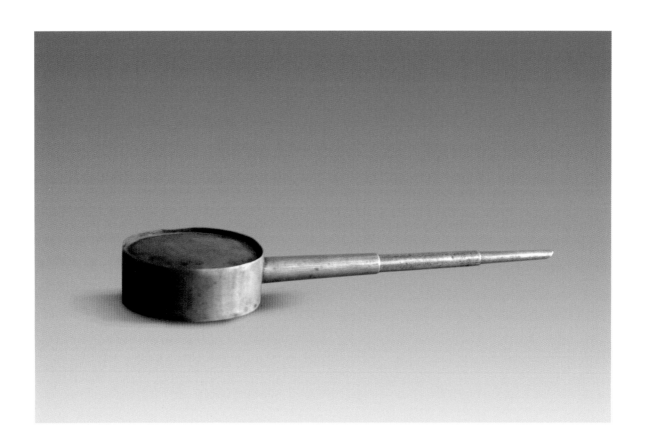

药鼓

民国时期

铜质

直径 4.5 厘米，长 15 厘米

Drum-like Medical Instrument

Republican Period

Copper

Diameter 4.5 cm/ Length 15 cm

吹药用具。体作圆鼓形，铜管多节。使用时，挤压圆鼓，可使药粉吹至病患处。由民间征集。

成都中医药大学中医药传统文化博物馆藏

The drum-like medical instrument was used for applying medicine. It is an instrument with a drum-like belly and a multi-section copper handle. When pressing the drum-like belly, the medicine powder can be blown to the affected part. It was collected from the folk.

Preserved in Museum of Traditional Chinese Medicine Culture, Chengdu University of Traditional Chinese Medicine

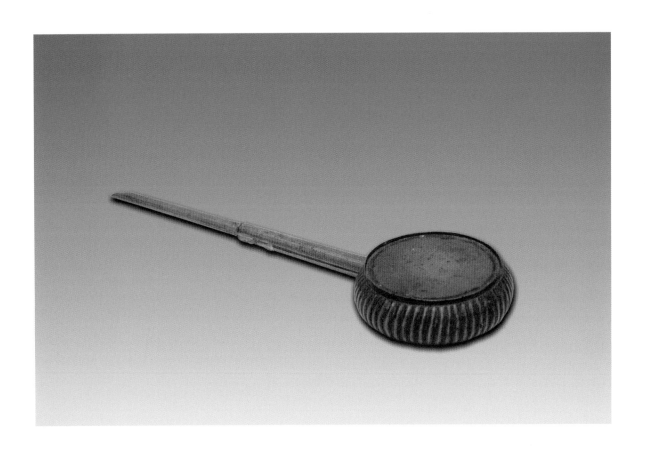

药鼓

民国时期

铜质

直径 4.5 厘米，长 15 厘米

Drum-like Medical Instrument

Republican Period

Copper

Diameter 4.5 cm/ Length 15 cm

吹药用具。体作圆鼓形，铜管多节。使用时，挤压圆鼓，可使药粉吹至病患处。由民间征集。

成都中医药大学中医药传统文化博物馆藏

The drum-like medical instrument was used for applying medicine. It is an instrument with a drum-like belly and a multi-section copper handle. When pressing the drum-like belly, the medicine powder can be blown to the affected part. It was collected from the folk.

Preserved in Museum of Traditional Chinese Medicine Culture, Chengdu University of Traditional Chinese Medicine

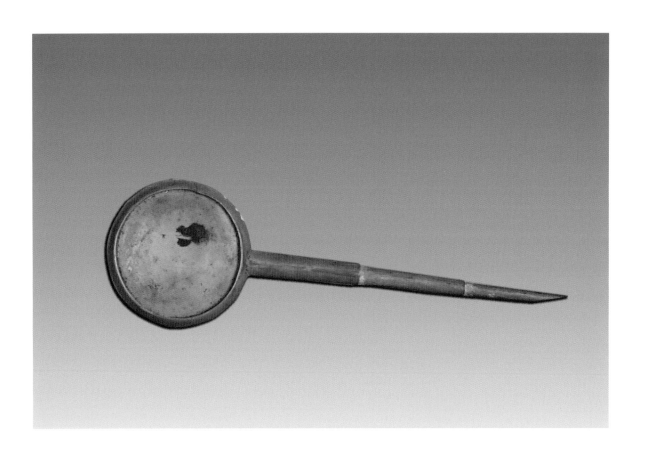

喷药粉器

民国时期

铜质

长 17 厘米，宽 5.3 厘米，厚 1.85 厘米

Medical Spray Tube

Republican Period

Copper

Length 17 cm/ Width 5.3 cm/ Thickness 1.85 cm

手鼓形，用于喷药。该藏表面光滑，工艺一般，喷管由三节构成，最前端口为斜口状。1959年入藏。保存基本完好。

中华医学会 / 上海中医药大学医史博物馆藏

The spray tube takes the shape of tambourine and is used for spraying medicine. With smooth surface, this three-part tube has a handle with an oblique opening, representing the mediocre workmanship. It was collected in 1959 and is still in good condition.

Preserved in Chinese Medical Association/ Museum of Chinese Medicine, Shanghai University of Traditional Chinese Medicine

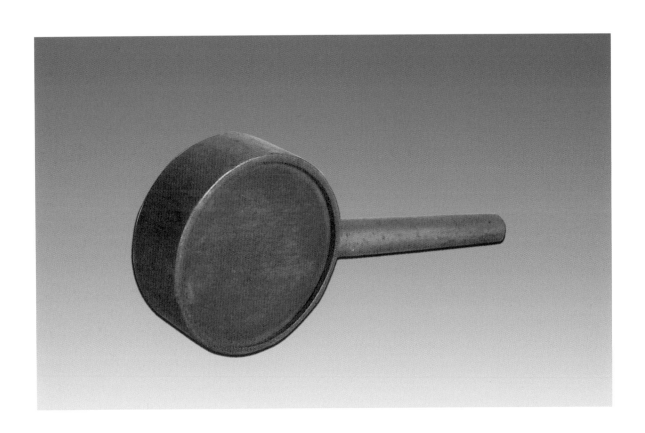

喷药粉器

民国时期

铜质

长 15.3 厘米，宽 4.4 厘米，厚 1.7 厘米

Medical Spray Tube

Republican Period

Copper

Length 15.3 cm/ Width 4.4 cm/ Thickness 1.7 cm

手鼓形，用于喷药。该藏表面光滑，工艺一般，喷管由二节构成，最前端口为斜口状。1959年入藏。保存基本完好。

中华医学会 / 上海中医药大学医史博物馆藏

The spray tube takes the shape of tambourine and is used for spraying medicine. With smooth surface, this two-part tube has a handle with an oblique opening, representing the mediocre workmanship. It was collected in 1959 and is still in good condition.

Preserved in Chinese Medical Association/ Museum of Chinese Medicine, Shanghai University of Traditional Chinese Medicine

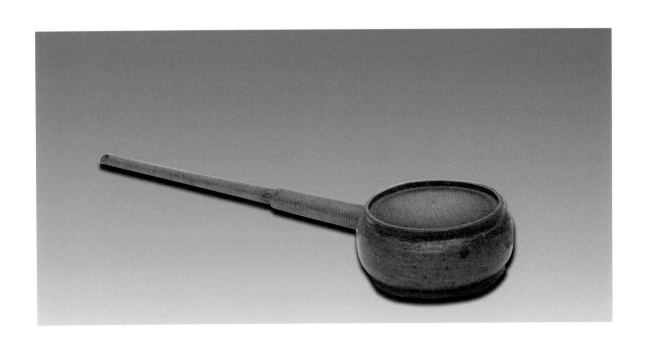

药鼓

民国时期

铜质

直径 3.5 厘米，长 16 厘米

吹药用具。体作圆鼓形，铜管多节。使用时，挤压圆鼓，可使药粉吹至病患处。由民间征集。

成都中医药大学中医药传统文化博物馆藏

Drum-like Medical Instrument

Republican Period

Copper

Diameter 3.5 cm/ Length 16 cm

The drum-like medical instrument was used for applying medicine. It is an instrument with a drum-like belly and a multi-section copper handle. When pressing the drum-like belly, the medicine powder can be blown to the affected part. It was collected from the folk.

Preserved in Museum of Traditional Chinese Medicine Culture, Chengdu University of Traditional Chinese Medicine

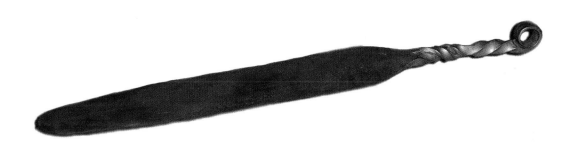

铜膏药刀

民国时期

铜质

长 26.5 厘米，宽 3.1 厘米，重 15 克

麻花状把，舌状刀。医疗器具。完整无损。

陕西医史博物馆藏

Copper Medical Plaster Knife

Republican Period

Copper

Length 26.5 cm/ Width 3.1 cm/ Weight 15 g

The plaster knife has a braided handle and a tongue-shaped blade. This medical instrument is still intact.

Preserved in Shaanxi Museum of Medical History

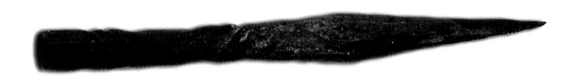

刀

民国时期

铁质

长 16 厘米

手术用具。由民间征集。

成都中医药大学中医药传统文化博物馆藏

Knife

Republican Period

Iron

Length 16 cm

The knife is a surgical instrument and was collected from the folk.

Preserved in Museum of Traditional Chinese Medicine Culture, Chengdu University of Traditional Chinese Medicine

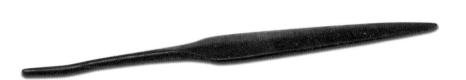

刀

民国时期

铁质

长 11.5 厘米

手术用具。由民间征集。

成都中医药大学中医药传统文化博物馆藏

Knife

Republican Period

Iron

Length 11.5 cm

The knife is a tool for operation. It was collected from the folk.

Preserved in Museum of Traditional Chinese Medicine Culture, Chengdu University of Traditional Chinese Medicine

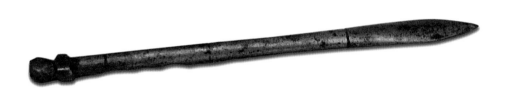

刀

民国时期

铜质

长 8.4 厘米

手术用具。由民间征集。

成都中医药大学中医药传统文化博物馆藏

Knife

Republican Period

Copper

Length 8.4 cm

The knife is a surgical instrument and was collected from the folk.

Preserved in Museum of Traditional Chinese Medicine Culture, Chengdu University of Traditional Chinese Medicine

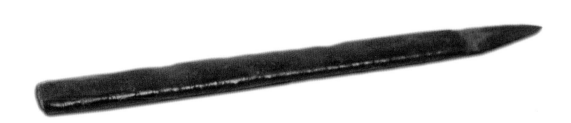

刀

民国时期

铁质

长 9.2 厘米

外科手术用具。由民间征集。

成都中医药大学中医药传统文化博物馆藏

Knife

Republican Period

Iron

Length 9.2 cm

The knife is a surgical instrument and was collected from the folk.

Preserved in Museum of Traditional Chinese Medicine Culture, Chengdu University of Traditional Chinese Medicine

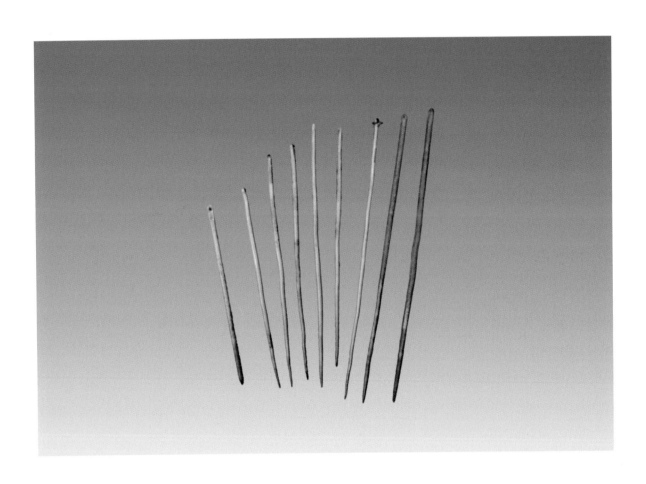

银九针

民国时期

银质

直径 1.3 厘米，长 0.3~10.7 厘米

Silver "Nine Needles"

Republican Period

Silver

Diameter 1.3 cm/ Length 0.3–10.7 cm

医用器具，一套 9 枚。此套银制九针是九针
发展过程中比较成熟阶段的产物，传承了明
清风格的民国针具。

张雅宗藏

Consisting of nine silver needles, this set of
medical appliance of Republic China Period
has inherited the style of the Ming and Qing
Dynasties and demonstrated the mature
development of "Nine Needles" (a set of ancient
traditional Chinese medical instruments) at that
time.

Collected by Zhang Yazong

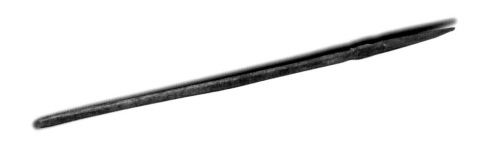

针

民国时期

铁质

长 13 厘米

手术用具。由民间征集。

成都中医药大学中医药传统文化博物馆藏

Needle

Republican Period

Iron

Length 13 cm

The needle is a surgical instrument and was collected from the folk.

Preserved in Museum of Traditional Chinese Medicine Culture, Chengdu University of Traditional Chinese Medicine

针

民国时期

铜质

长 11 厘米

由民间征集。

成都中医药大学中医药传统文化博物馆藏

Needle

Republican Period

Copper

Length 11 cm

The needle was collected from the folk.

Preserved in Museum of Traditional Chinese Medicine Culture, Chengdu University of Traditional Chinese Medicine

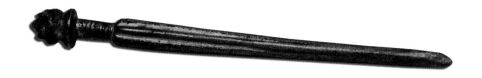

针

民国时期

铜质

长 9.5 厘米

尾部有花朵状装饰。由民间征集。

成都中医药大学中医药传统文化博物馆藏

Needle

Republican Period

Copper

Length 9.5 cm

The needle is engraved with flower-shaped pattern at the tail and it was collected from the folk.

Preserved in Museum of Traditional Chinese Medicine Culture, Chengdu University of Traditional Chinese Medicine

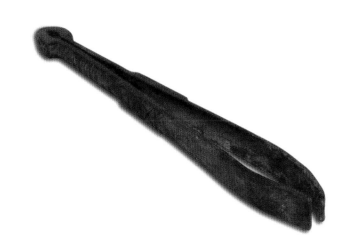

镊子

民国时期

铁质

长 8.4 厘米

手术用具。由民间征集。

成都中医药大学中医药传统文化博物馆藏

Tweezers

Republican Period

Iron

Length 8.4 cm

The tweezers is a surgical instrument and was collected from the folk.

Preserved in Museum of Traditional Chinese Medicine Culture, Chengdu University of Traditional Chinese Medicine

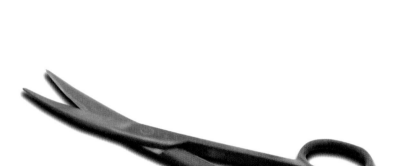

剪

民国时期

铁质

长 14 厘米

手术用具。由民间征集。

成都中医药大学中医药传统文化博物馆藏

Scissors

Republican Period

Iron

Length 14 cm

The scissors is a surgical instrument and was collected from the folk.

Preserved in Museum of Traditional Chinese Medicine Culture, Chengdu University of Traditional Chinese Medicine

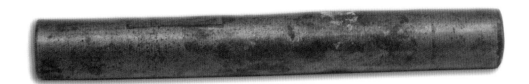

针筒

民国时期

铜质

口径 1.5 厘米，长 13.5 厘米

由民间征集。

成都中医药大学中医药传统文化博物馆藏

Syringe

Republican Period

Copper

Mouth Diameter 1.5 cm/ Length 13.5 cm

The syringe was collected from the folk.

Preserved in Museum of Traditional Chinese Medicine Culture, Chengdu University of Traditional Chinese Medicine

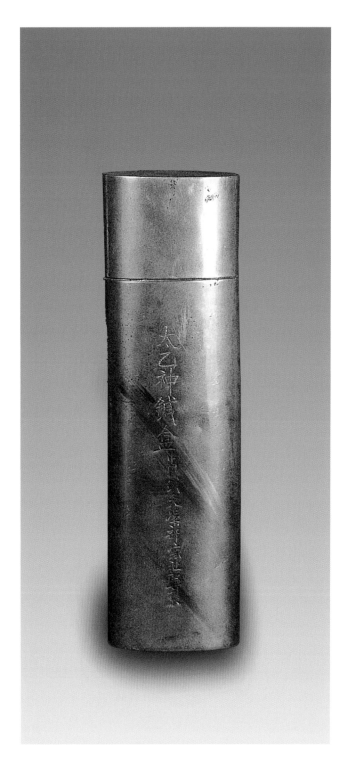

"太乙神针"铜藏针筒

民国时期

铜质

底径 6.2 厘米，长 20.5 厘米

Copper Cylinder of "Taiyi Miraculous Needles"

Republican Period

Copper

Bottom Diameter 6.2 cm/ Length 20.5 cm

椭圆形。正面刻有"太乙神针盒 中国针灸学研究社监制"字样。该社系承淡庵创办。

上海中医药博物馆藏

The needle cylinder is oval-shaped with the inscription meaning "Taiyi Miraculous needles, made by China Acupuncture and Moxibustion Society" on the front. The society was founded by Cheng Dan'an, a famous Chinese doctor.

Preserved in Shanghai Museum of Traditional Chinese Medicine

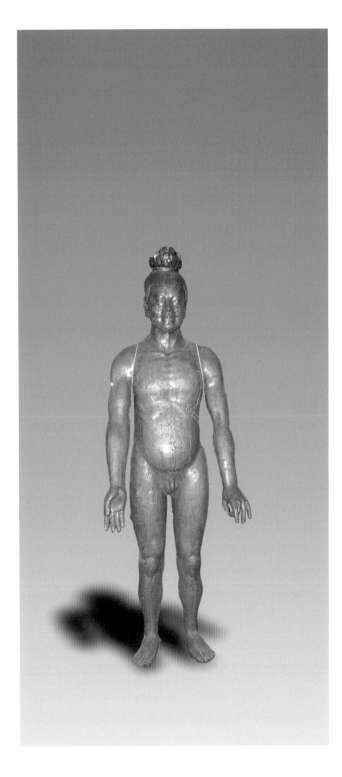

针灸铜人

现代

铜质

高 170 厘米

Copper Acupuncture Status

Modern Times

Copper

Height 170 cm

该仿制品为一成年男子正面站立形象，体表标明经络循行路线及腧穴位置、名称等。教学陈列品。完整无损。1984 年入藏，江苏省新医学院仿制。

陕西医史博物馆藏

Standing facing the front, the copper acupuncture status demonstrates the channel distribution and the acupuncture points. This teaching exhibit was collected in 1984 and is still intact. It is a duplicate made by the New Medical College of Jiangsu Province (now Nanjing Medical University).

Preserved in Shaanxi Museum of Medical History

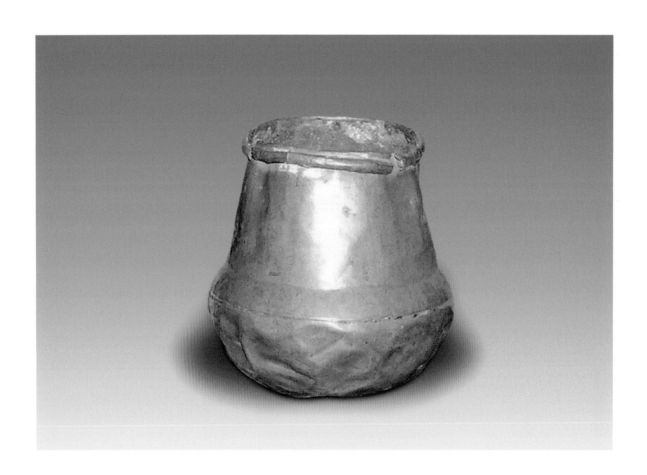

拔火罐

民国时期

铜质

口径 3.4 厘米，通高 5 厘米，重 23 克

Cupping Glass

Republican Period

Copper

Mouth Diameter 3.4 cm/ Height 5 cm/ Weight 23 g

口沿外卷，斜颈，圆腹，圆底，表面不平。医药
器具。口沿有残。内蒙古自治区包头市征集。

陕西医史博物馆藏

The cupping glass, a medical appliance, has an
outward-rolled mouth, an oblique neck, a round
belly, a round bottom and a rough surface. The
mouth is somewhat damaged. It was collected
in Baotou City, the Inner Mongolia Autonomous
Region.

Preserved in Shaanxi Museum of Medical History

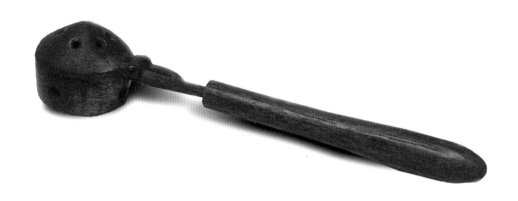

温灸器

民国时期

铜质

长 23 厘米

木柄便于手持。由民间征集。

成都中医药大学中医药传统文化博物馆藏

Moxa Burner

Republican Period

Copper

Length 23 cm

The moxa burner has a convenient wooden handle. It was collected from the folk.

Preserved in Museum of Traditional Chinese Medicine Culture, Chengdu University of Traditional Chinese Medicine

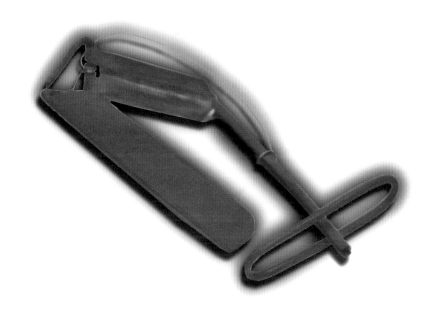

灸条夹

民国时期

铜质

长 6 厘米

由民间征集。

成都中医药大学中医药传统文化博物馆藏

Clamp for Moxa Stick

Republican Period

Copper

Length 6 cm

It was collected from the folk.

Preserved in Museum of Traditional Chinese Medicine Culture, Chengdu University of Traditional Chinese Medicine

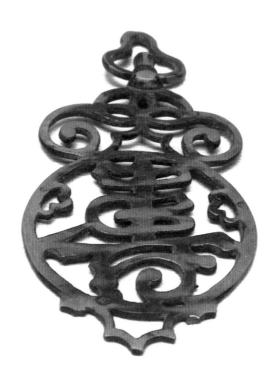

佩饰

民国时期

铜质

长 12 厘米

由镂空的"寿"字和枝叶组成。由民间征集。

成都中医药大学中医药传统文化博物馆藏

Accessory

Republican Period

Copper

Length 12 cm

The accessory consists of a hollow Chinese character " 寿 " (Shou, meaning longevity) and other patterns of branches and leaves. It was collected from the folk.

Preserved in Museum of Traditional Chinese Medicine Culture, Chengdu University of Traditional Chinese Medicine

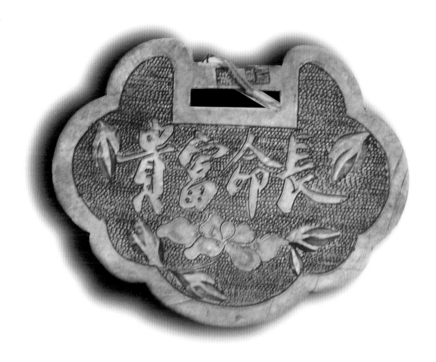

佩饰

民国时期

银质

长 5.7 厘米

镌刻 "长命富贵" 四字和枝叶纹。由民间征集。

成都中医药大学中医药传统文化博物馆藏

Accessory

Republican Period

Silver

Length 5.7 cm

The accessory is engraved with four Chinese characters reading "Chang Ming Fu Gui" (means longevity and wealth) and other patterns of branches and leaves. It was collected from the folk.

Preserved in Museum of Traditional Chinese Medicine Culture, Chengdu University of Traditional Chinese Medicine

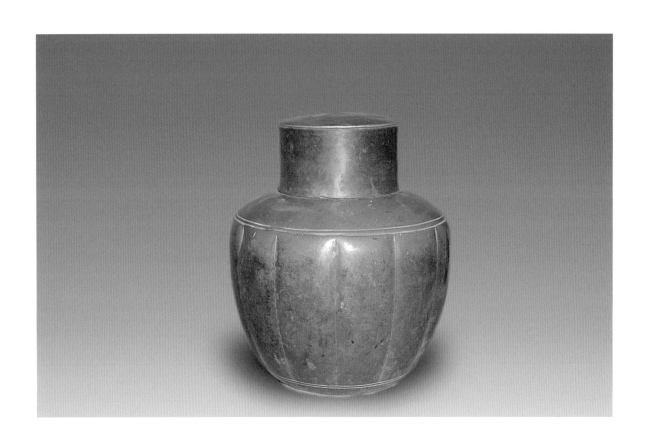

锡罐

近代

锡质

口径 10.1 厘米，底径 10.5 厘米，通高 21.2 厘米，重 1900 克

Tin Pot

Modern Times

Tin

Mouth Diameter 10.1 cm/ Bottom Diameter 10.5 cm/ Height 21.2 cm/ Weight 1,900 g

子母口，圆肩，平底，底有"道口聚盛"字
样。盛贮器。完整无损。聚盛锡店河南滑县
道口生产规模较大。锡罐具有良好的密闭性
和保鲜功能，可避免中药和茶叶营养流失、
变味、变色。明·周高起："纯锡为五金之母，
以制茶铫，能益水德，沸亦声耳。"

陕西医史博物馆藏

The tin pot has two matching mouths, a round shoulder and a flat bottom engraved with the Chinese characters reading "Dao Kou Ju Sheng". It was used as a container. It is intact. Jusheng Tin shop in Taokou Town, Huaxian County, Henan Province is well-known for its massive production of tin pots. Tin pots have good tightness, and can best retain the freshness of Chinese medicine and tea by preventing the nutrients from changing in flavor or color. Zhou Gaoqi in Ming Dynasty once said that "pure tin is the mother of the five metals. Once made into a teapot, it helps the water to be better. Even the boiling water will also sound good."

Preserved in Shaanxi Museum of Medical History

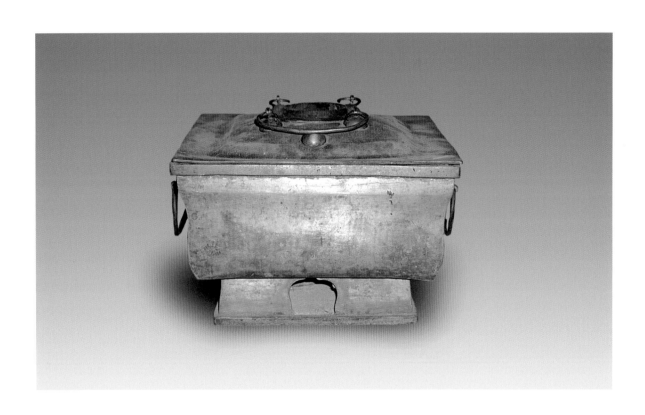

锡火锅

近代

锡质

口径 22 厘米，底径 16 厘米，通高 15.5 厘米，
重 3750 克

方形，带盖，火锅样，盖有六个乳钉。炊器。
完整无损。

陕西医史博物馆藏

Tin Stove

Modern Times

Tin

Mouth Diameter 22 cm/ Bottom Diameter 16 cm/
Height 15.5 cm/ Weight 3,750 g

The squared-shaped tin stove has a cover. The
cover has six nipples on it. It was used as a
cooking vessel and remains intact.

Preserved in Shaanxi Museum of Medical History

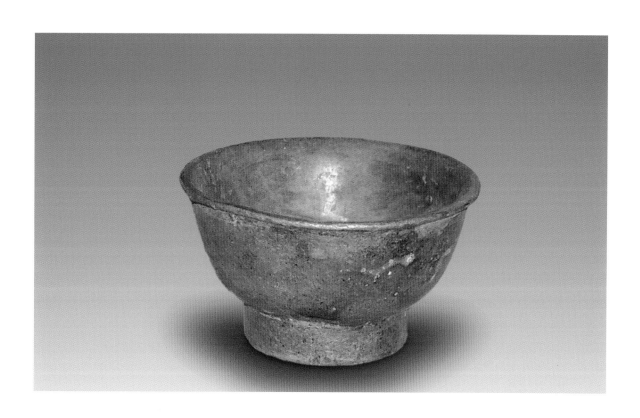

铜酒杯

民国时期

铜质

口径 4 厘米，底径 2 厘米，通高 2.2 厘米，重 50 克

敞口，斜腹，圈足。酒器。完整无损。

陕西医史博物馆藏

Copper Wine Cup

Republican Period

Copper

Mouth Diameter 4 cm/ Bottom Diameter 2 cm/ Height 2.2 cm/ Weight 50 g

The cup has an open mouth, an oblique belly and a ring-like foot. It was used as a drinking vessel and remains intact.

Preserved in Shaanxi Museum of Medical History

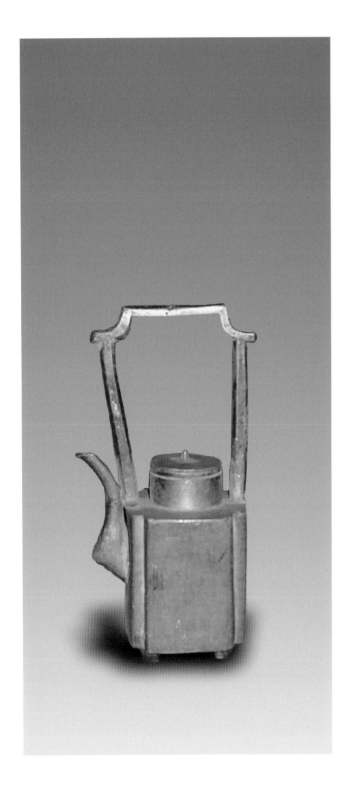

小锡壶

民国时期

锡质

口径 3.5 厘米，底径 6 厘米，通高 18 厘米，
重 500 克

Small Tin Pot

Republican Period

Tin

Mouth Diameter 3.5 cm/ Bottom Diameter 6 cm/

Height 18 cm/Weight 500 g

亚字形壶，高提梁，有一水流。贮水器。完整无损。陕西省咸阳市秦都区征集。

陕西医史博物馆藏

The pot is shaped like a Chinese character "亚" with a high hoop handle and a spout. It was used as a water container and remains intact. The pot was collected in Qindu District, Xianyang City, Shaanxi Province.

Preserved in Shaanxi Museum of Medical History

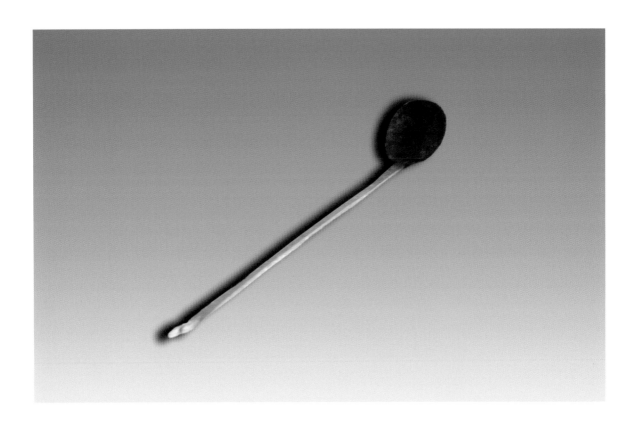

匙

近代

铁质

长 12.5 厘米

由民间征集。

　　　　成都中医药大学中医药传统文化博物馆藏

Spoon

Modern Times

Iron

Length 12.5 cm

The spoon was collected from the folk.

Preserved in Museum of Traditional Chinese Medicine Culture, Chengdu University of Traditional Chinese Medicine

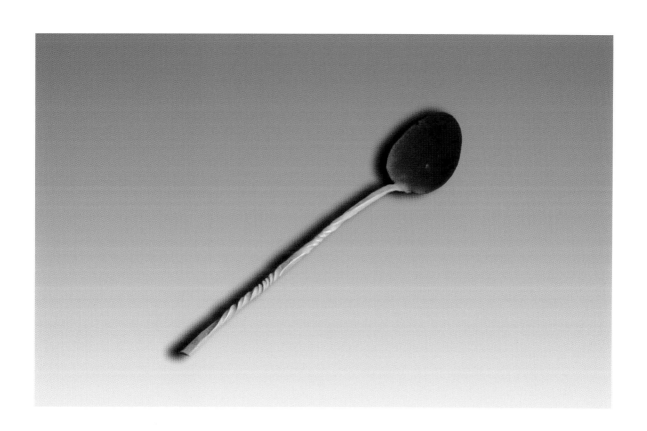

匙

Spoon

近代

铁质

长 12 厘米

由民间征集。

　　成都中医药大学中医药传统文化博物馆藏

Modern Times

Iron

Length 12 cm

The spoon was collected from the folk.

Preserved in Museum of Traditional Chinese
Medicine Culture, Chengdu University of Traditional
Chinese Medicine

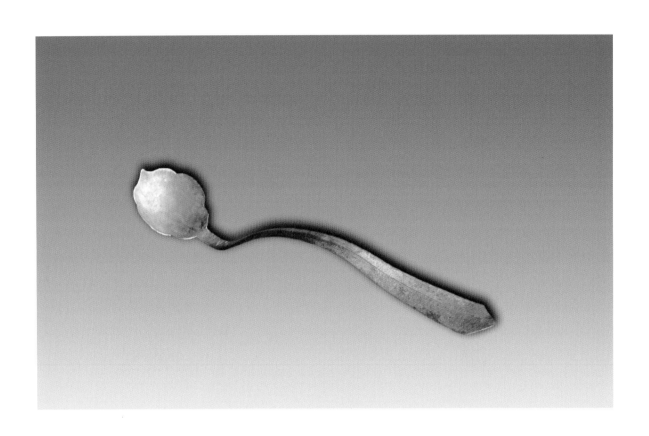

匙

民国时期

铜质

长 15 厘米

该匙柄为圆弧形，匙心为葵瓣纹。由民间征集。

成都中医药大学中医药传统文化博物馆藏

Spoon

Republican Period

Copper

Length 15 cm

The spoon has an arc handle and a head like a petal of sunflower. It was collected from the folk.

Preserved in Museum of Traditional Chinese Medicine Culture, Chengdu University of Traditional Chinese Medicine

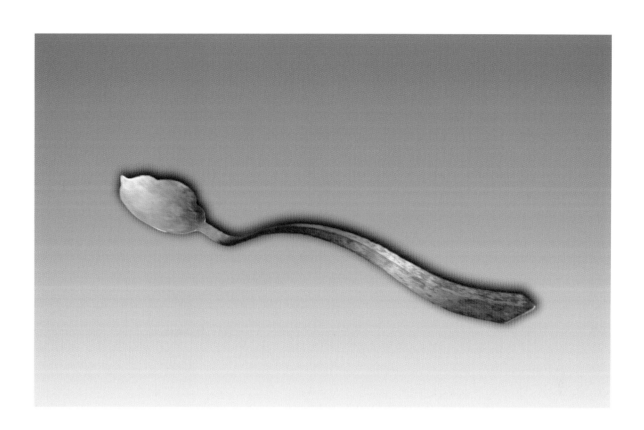

匙

Spoon

民国时期

铜质

长 16 厘米

匙柄为圆弧形，匙心为葵瓣纹。由民间征集。

成都中医药大学中医药传统文化博物馆藏

Republican Period

Copper

Length 16 cm

The spoon has an arc handle and a head like a petal of sunflower. It was collected from the folk.

Preserved in Museum of Traditional Chinese Medicine Culture, Chengdu University of Traditional Chinese Medicine

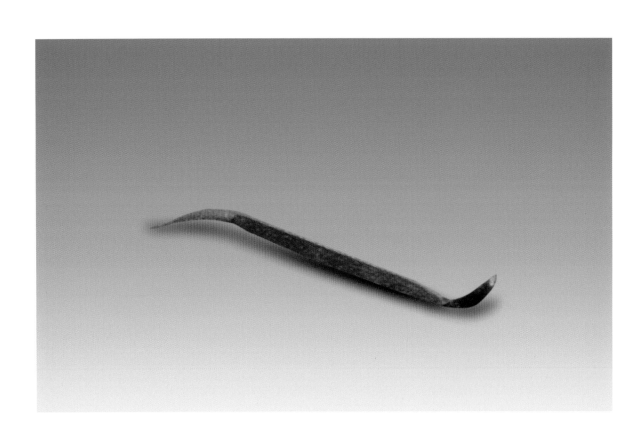

勺

民国时期

铁质

长 17 厘米

一端为尖状，可两用。由民间征集。

　　成都中医药大学中医药传统文化博物馆藏

Spoon

Republican Period

Iron

Length 17 cm

The spoon has a pointed handle end and serves two purposes. It was collected from the folk.

Preserved in Museum of Traditional Chinese Medicine Culture, Chengdu University of Traditional Chinese Medicine

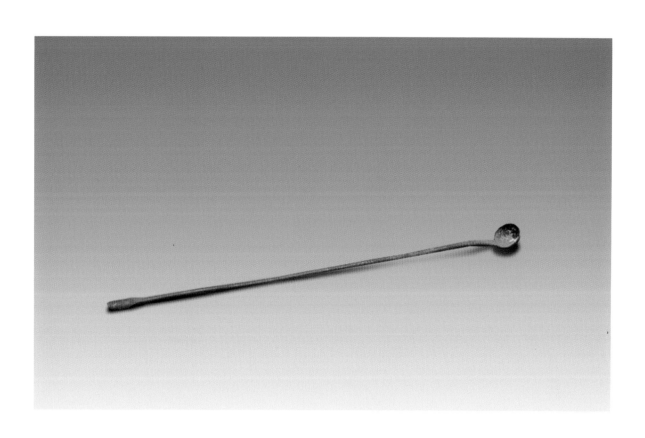

匙

Spoon

民国时期

铁质

长 21 厘米

由民间征集。

成都中医药大学中医药传统文化博物馆藏

Republican Period

Iron

Length 21 cm

The spoon was collected from the folk.

Preserved in Museum of Traditional Chinese Medicine Culture, Chengdu University of Traditional Chinese Medicine

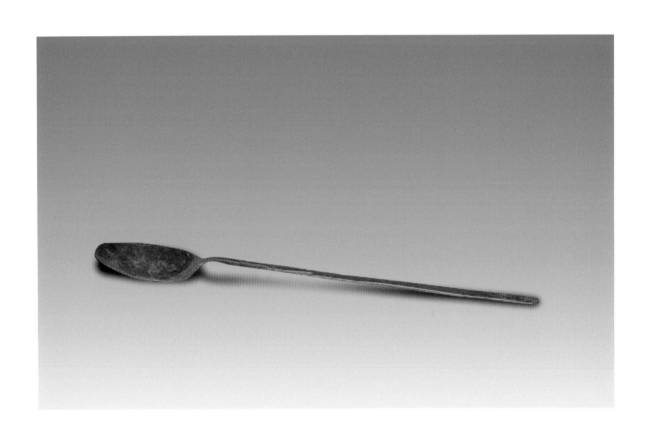

铜勺

民国时期

铜质

长 20 厘米，宽 3.6 厘米，重 50 克

小勺状，柄为长扁形。生活用具。完整无损。

陕西医史博物馆藏

Copper Spoon

Republican Period

Copper

Length 20 cm/ Width 3.6 cm/ Weight 50 g

The copper spoon is small with a long flat handle.
It was used as a life utensil, and was collected from
the folk.

Preserved in Shaanxi Museum of Medical History

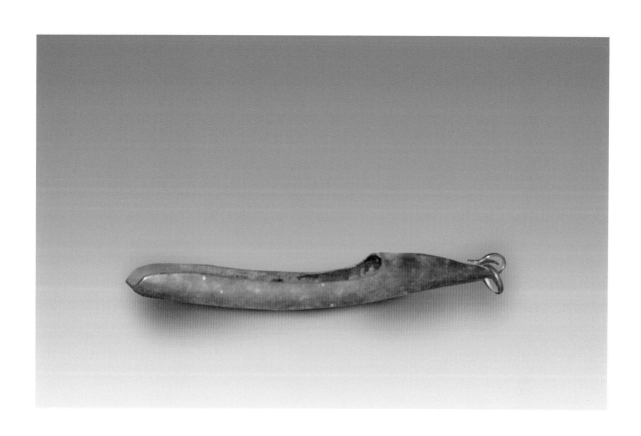

铜马勺

民国时期

铜质

长 32 厘米，宽 3 厘米，重 350 克

呈船形，右头上翘并有一环。生活用器。完整无损。内蒙古历史博物馆调拨。

陕西医史博物馆藏

Copper Ladle

Republican Period

Copper

Length 32 cm/ Width 3 cm/ Weight 350 g

The spoon is boat-shaped with a ring on the right end. It was used as a life utensil and remains intact. It was transferred from Inner Mongolia History Museum.

Preserved in Shaanxi Museum of Medical History

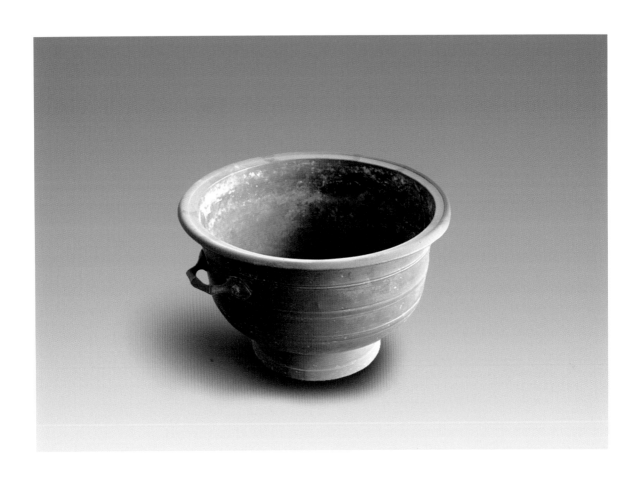

洗

民国时期

铜质

口径 33 厘米，高 20 厘米

Washer

Republican Period

Copper

Mouth Diameter 33 cm/ Height 20 cm

直腹，圈足，腹上有三道旋纹，双耳。洗面
用具。由民间征集。

　　成都中医药大学中医药传统文化博物馆藏

The spoon has an straight belly, a ring-like
foot and two ears. There are three revolved
lines around the belly. It was used as a washing
utensil and was collected from the folk.
Preserved in Museum of Traditional Chinese
Medicine Culture, Chengdu University of Traditional
Chinese Medicine

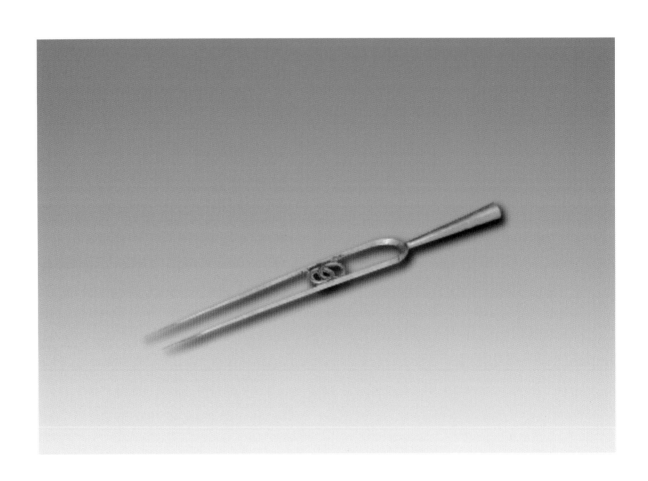

铜叉

民国时期

黄铜质

长 12 厘米，宽 1.2 厘米，重 25 克

Copper Fork

Republican Period

Copper

Length 12 cm/ Width 1.2 cm/ Weight 25 g

两股叉状，两叉之间有两套环。生活用器。

完整无损。内蒙古征集。

陕西医史博物馆藏

The two-tined fork has two rings between the

tines. It was used as a life utensil and remains

intact. It was collected in Inner Mongolia.

Preserved in Shaanxi Museum of Medical History

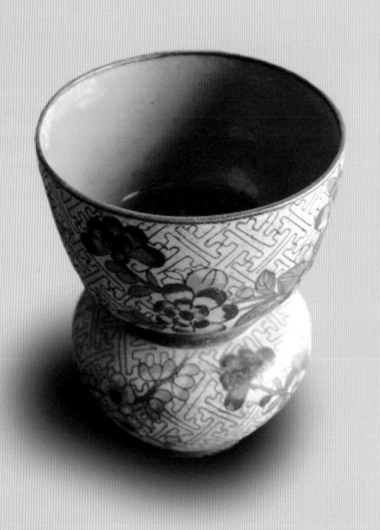

唾盂

民国时期

铜胎掐丝

口径 7.7 厘米，底径 4.0 厘米，高 10.2 厘米

景泰蓝制作，分上、下两层，均饰有文房四宝及花卉等图案，上部稍大呈锥形，下部为直口，鼓腹，底部微敛，圈足。此类唾盂多放于书案或床头，制作精细，图案与环境比较协调。由民间征集。

成都中医药大学中医药传统文化博物馆藏

Spittoon

Republican Period

Copper Padding with Thread Weaving

Mouth Diameter 7.7 cm/ Bottom Diameter 4.0 cm/ Height 10.2 cm

The spittoon is made of cloisonne. It has two parts with designs of four treasures of study (writing brush, ink stick, ink slab and paper), flowers and others on it. The top is bigger and cone-shaped. The base has a straight mouth, a swelling belly, a tightened bottom and a ring-like foot. This kind of spittoon is always put on a writing desk or by the head of a bed. It was finely produced with patterns going well with the surroundings. It was collected from the folk.

Preserved in Museum of Traditional Chinese Medicine Culture, Chengdu University of Traditional Chinese Medicine

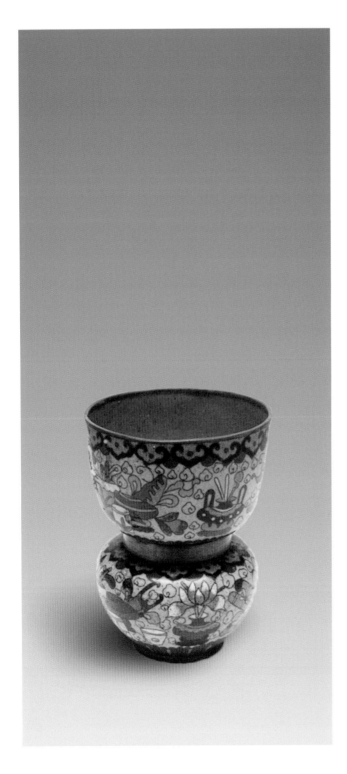

唾盂

民国时期

铜胎掐丝

口径 7.5 厘米，底径 3.7 厘米，高 9.6 厘米

Spittoon

Republican Period

Copper Padding with Thread Weaving

Mouth Diameter 7.5 cm/ Bottom Diameter 3.7 cm/

Height 9.6 cm

景泰蓝制作，上、下两层，均饰有花卉纹，上部呈钵形，下部为直口，鼓腹，平底，圈足。由民间征集。

成都中医药大学中医药传统文化博物馆藏

The spittoon is made of cloisonne. It has two parts with designs of flowers on it. The top is bowl-shaped. The base has a straight mouth, a swelling belly, a flat bottom and a ring-like foot. It was collected from the folk.

Preserved in Museum of Traditional Chinese Medicine Culture, Chengdu University of Traditional Chinese Medicine

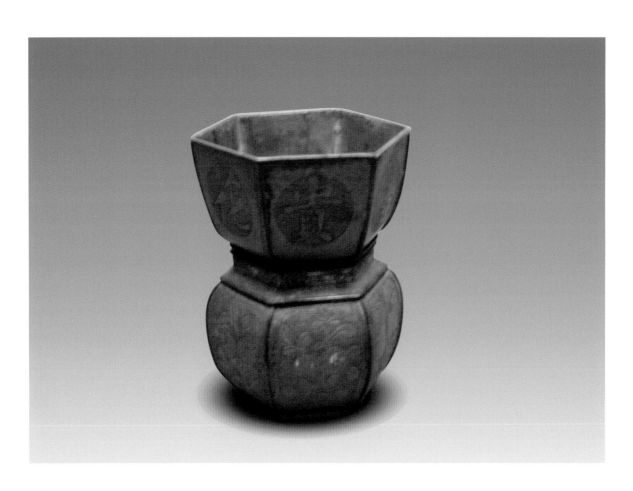

唾盂

民国时期

锡质

口径 6 厘米，底径 3.7 厘米，高 8.8 厘米

Spittoon

Republican Period

Tin

Mouth Diameter 6 cm/ Bottom Diameter 3.7 cm/ Height 8.8 cm

六边瓜棱形，分上、下两层，上部为钵形，下部为鼓形，圈足上下均刻有纹饰图案，上部饰有"花笑蝴蝶富贵"六字，下部为花卉纹。由民间征集。

成都中医药大学中医药传统文化博物馆藏

The spittoon is hexagonal, prismatic and melon-shaped. It has two parts, the bowl-shaped top and the drum-shaped bottom. The ring-like foot has patterns on each end, with the top end engraved with the Chinese characters reading "Hua Xiao Hu Die Fu Gui" (smiling flowers, butterflies and wealth) and the bottom end decorated with patterns of flowers. It was collected from the folk.

Preserved in Museum of Traditional Chinese Medicine Culture, Chengdu University of Traditional Chinese Medicine

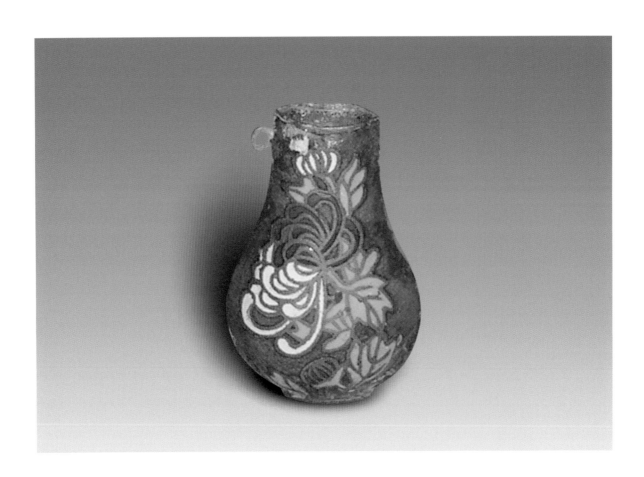

景泰蓝小蓝瓶

民国时期

铜质

口径 1.1 厘米，底径 1 厘米，通高 3.5 厘米，重 20 克

Small Cloisonne Vase

Republican Period

Copper

Mouth Diameter 1.1 cm/ Bottom Diameter 1 cm/ Height 3.5 cm/ Weight 20 g

扁口，口上有双耳，扁腹，平底，腹上有花纹。
工艺品。完整无损。

陕西医史博物馆藏

The vase has a flat mouth, two ears around the
mouth, a flattened belly and a flat bottom. The
belly has decorative patterns on it. The vase is a
well-preserved craft.
Preserved in Shaanxi Museum of Medical History

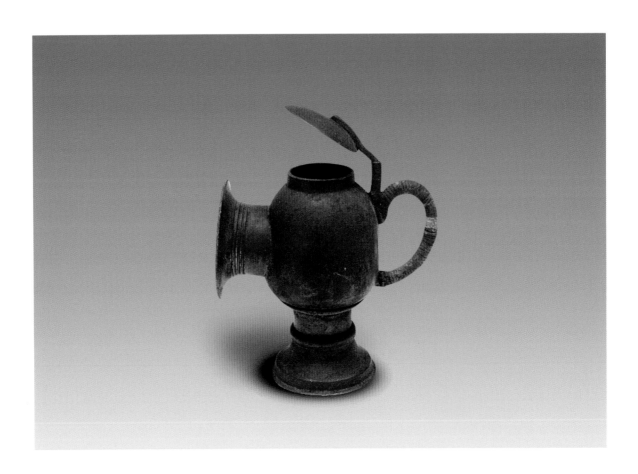

灭蚊灯

民国时期

锡质

上口径 3.5 厘米，侧端口径 6.2 厘米，底径 5.9 厘米，宽 11 厘米

Mosquito Killer Lamp

Republican Period

Tin

Upper Mouth Diameter 3.5 cm/ Side Mouth Diameter 6.2 cm/ Bottom Diameter 5.9 cm/ Width 11 cm

器形完好，分上、下两部分，下方盛燃油，内有灯芯，上方顶端开圆口，腹部侧端喇叭口形成负压，可将蚊虫吸入烧死。上端口部有一盖，腹部有一把手，底部有"昌泰鸿用包造"铭。民间征集。

成都中医药大学中医药传统文化博物馆藏

The lamp is intact and has two parts. The lower half can be filled with fuel oil and has wick in it. The upper half has a round mouth on the top. The flared mouth on the side of the belly forms negative pressure and helps burn the mosquitoes through inhalation. There is a cover over the upper mouth and a handle on the belly. The bottom is engraved with the inscription reading "Chang Tai Hong Yong Bao Zao" (place of production). It was collected from the folk.
Preserved in Museum of Traditional Chinese Medicine Culture, Chengdu University of Traditional Chinese Medicine

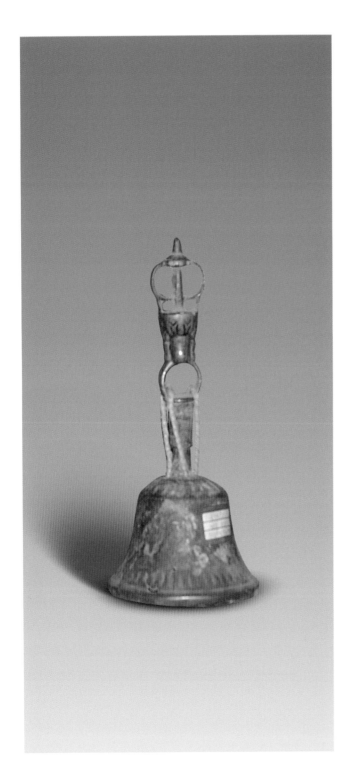

铜铃

革命战争时期

铜质

口径5厘米，底径9厘米，通高21.5厘米，重450克

手摇铃，喇叭口，活动手柄。生活用器。完整无损。陕西省延安市文化馆征集。

陕西医史博物馆藏

Copper Bell

Revolution Period

Copper

Mouth Diameter 5 cm/ Bottom Diameter 9 cm/ Height 21.5 cm/ Weight 450 g

The hand bell has a flared mouth and a movable handle. It is a well-preserved life appliance, collected from Yan'an Cultural Center of Shaanxi Province.

Preserved in Shaanxi Museum of Medical History

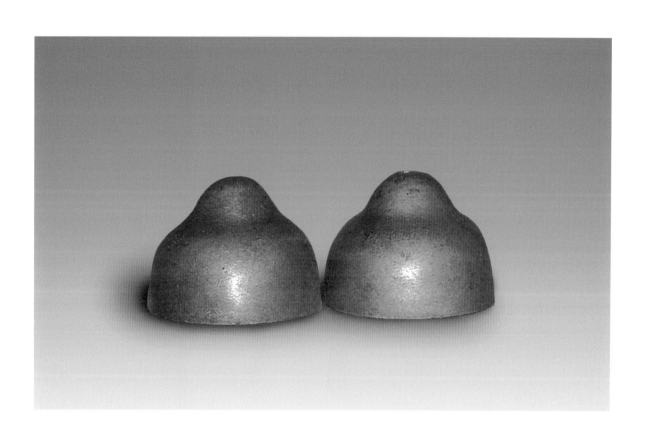

铜铃（甩子）

近代

铜质

口径 1.5 厘米，底径 5 厘米，通高 4 厘米，重
250 克

铃铛形，草帽状。民族乐器。完整无损。

陕西医史博物馆藏

Copper Bell (Hollow Swage)

Modern Times

Copper

Mouth Diameter 1.5 cm/ Bottom Diameter 5 cm/
Height 4 cm/ Weight 250 g

The bell is in the shape of straw hat. It was used as
a folk musical instrument and remains intact.

Preserved in Shaanxi Museum of Medical History

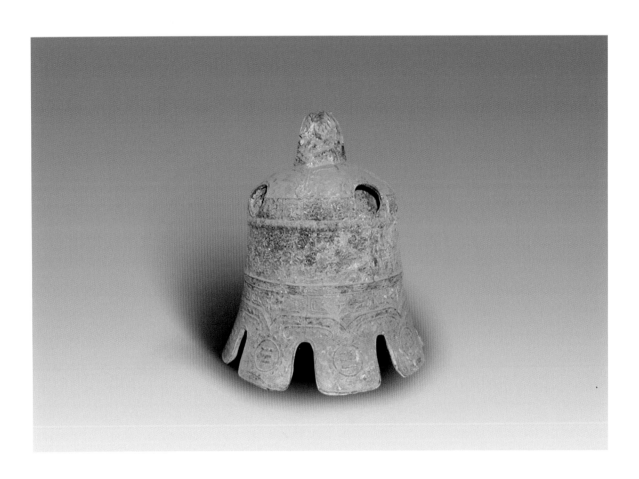

铁钟

清

铁质

上口径 31.5 厘米，底径 46 厘米，通高 48 厘米

Iron Bell

Qing Dynasty

Iron

Upper Mouth Diameter 31.5 cm/ Bottom Diameter 46 cm/ Height 48 cm

传统钟形，底部八瓣为八卦图，腹有铭文，肩部开有四个泛音孔，顶部有一悬钮，光绪元年四月造。宗教器物。完整无损。陕西省渭南市白水县征集。

陕西医史博物馆藏

The bell is in the traditional shape. The eight parts of the bottom are in the patterns of Eight Diagrams. There are inscriptions on the belly, four sound holes on the shoulder and a knob at the top. It was made in April, the first year of the reign of Emperor Guangxu and was used as a religious utensil, remaining intact. It was collected in Baishui County, Weinan City, Shaanxi Province.

Preserved in Shaanxi Museum of Medical History

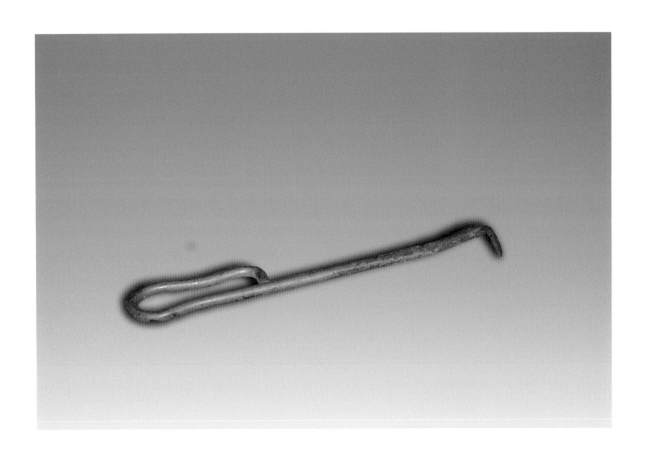

铜镰

现代

铜质

长 18 厘米，刀宽 0.3 厘米，重 50 克

头为镰刀状。生产工具。完整无损。

陕西医史博物馆藏

Copper Sickle

Modern Times

Copper

Length 18 cm/ Width 0.3 cm/ Weight 50 g

The head of the sickle is in the shape of reaping hook. It was used as an instrument of production and remains intact.

Preserved in Shaanxi Museum of Medical History

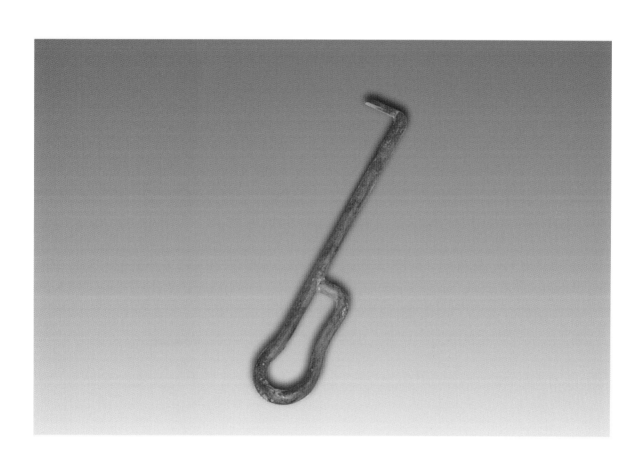

铜镰

现代

铜质

长 18 厘米，刀宽 0.5 厘米，重 50 克

头为镰刀状，把为圆形。生产工具。完整无损。

陕西医史博物馆藏

Copper Sickle

Modern Times

Copper

Length 18 cm/ Width 0.5 cm/ Weight 50 g

The head of the sickle is in the shape of reaping hook. The sickle has a round handle. It was used as an instrument of production and remains intact.

Preserved in Shaanxi Museum of Medical History

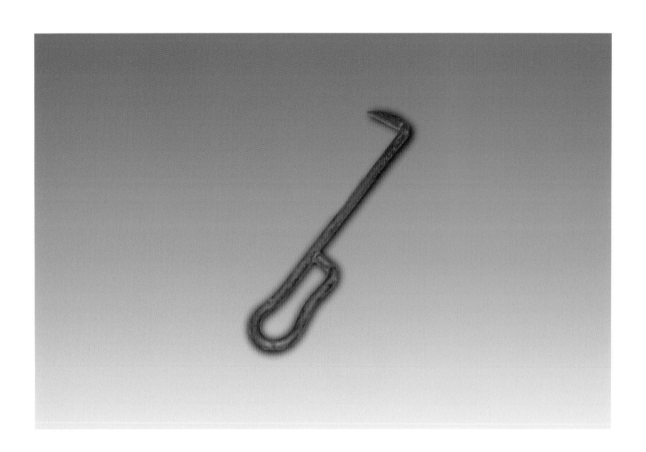

铜镰

现代

铜质

长 18 厘米，刀宽 0.8 厘米，重 50 克

头为镰刀状，刀把为圆形。生产工具。完整无损。

陕西医史博物馆藏

Copper Sickle

Modern Times

Copper

Length 18 cm/ Width 0.8 cm/ Weight 50 g

The head of the sickle is in the shape of reaping hook. The sickle has a round handle. It was used as an instrument of production and remains intact.

Preserved in Shaanxi Museum of Medical History

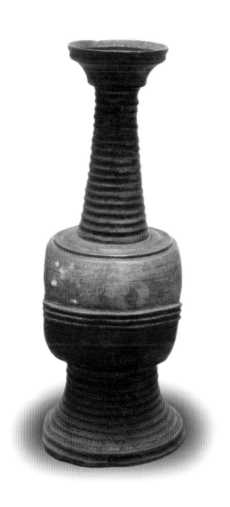

酒瓶

民国时期

铜质

高 24 厘米

盘口，竹节状颈，高圈足，是藏族地区盛酒用具。由民间征集。

成都中医药大学中医药传统文化博物馆藏

Wine Bottle

Republican Period

Copper

Height 24 cm

The bottle has a plate-shaped mouth, a neck with bamboo patterns and a high ring-like foot. It was used as a wine container in Tibetan area, and it was collected from the folk.

Preserved in Museum of Traditional Chinese Medicine Culture, Chengdu University of Traditional Chinese Medicine

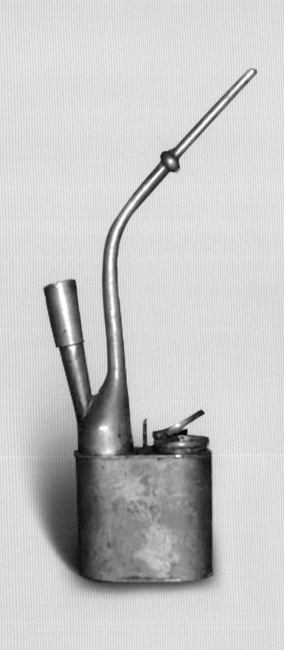

铜水烟袋

民国时期

铜质

口径 7.2 厘米，底径 7.2 厘米，通高 26.5 厘米，重 450 克

方形，左右两边为弧形，有浅浮雕松树、仙鹤图案，上部有两孔，长弯形烟嘴，底部有两圆孔。烟具。完整无损。

陕西医史博物馆藏

Copper Hookah

Republican Period

Copper

Mouth Diameter 7.2 cm/ Bottom Diameter 7.2 cm/ Height 26.5 cm/Weight 450 g

Its square body has two cambered sides with bas-relief of pine trees and red-crowned cranes on them. There are two holes on the top and a long curved cigarette holder and two round holes at the bottom. It was used as a smoking set and remains intact.

Preserved in Shaanxi Museum of Medical History

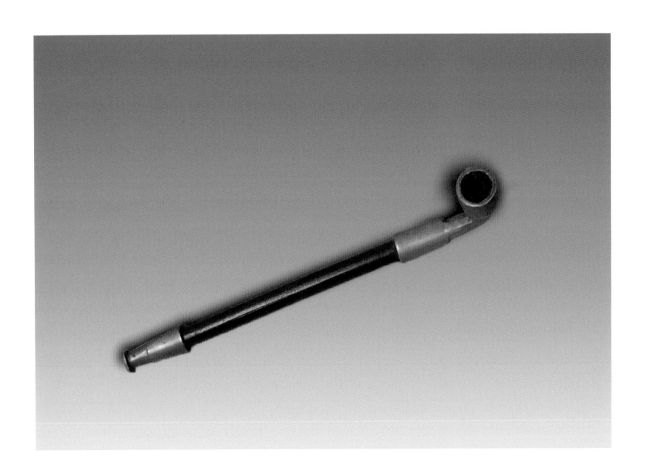

烟嘴

近现代

铜质木柄

烟杆直径 0.5 厘米，烟锅直径 1.1 厘米，通长 11.9 厘米

Tobacco Pipe

Modern Times

Copper Head, Wood Handle

Diameter of the Tobacco Stem 0.5 cm/ Diameter of the Head of the Pipe 1.1 cm/ Length 11.9 cm

烟斗形，为烟具。该藏铜嘴、铜锅、木柄，
造型美观精巧，有使用痕迹。1955 年入藏。
保存基本完好。

中华医学会 / 上海中医药大学医史博物馆藏

The pipe was used as a smoking set. This
collection has a copper holder, a copper head
and a wooden handle. It shows attractive and
delicate appearance and has been used. It was
collected in 1955 and is still in good condition.
Preserved in Chinese Medical Association/
Museum of Chinese Medicine, Shanghai
University of Traditional Chinese Medicine

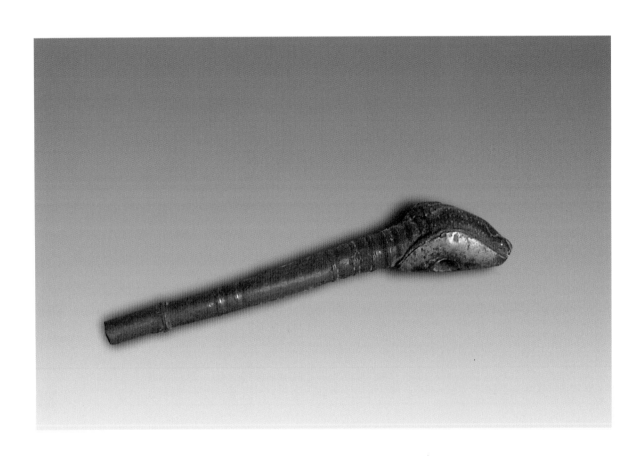

旱烟管

民国时期

铜质

长 14.15 厘米，宽 2 厘米

Tobacco Pipe

Republican Period

Copper

Length 14.15 cm/ Width 2 cm

烟斗形，为烟具。该藏表面光滑，工艺精细，

烟杆部刻饰竹节纹，头部加工精细，雕有花

卉及几何图案。1959年入藏。保存基本完好。

中华医学会 / 上海中医药大学医史博物馆藏

The tobacco pipe was used as a smoking set. This collection has a smooth surface and was made with fine craft. The pipe stem is engraved with the bamboo patterns. The head of the pipe is also delicate with engravings of flower patterns and geometric patterns. It was collected in 1959 and is still in good condition.

Preserved in Chinese Medical Association/ Museum of Chinese Medicine, Shanghai University of Traditional Chinese Medicine

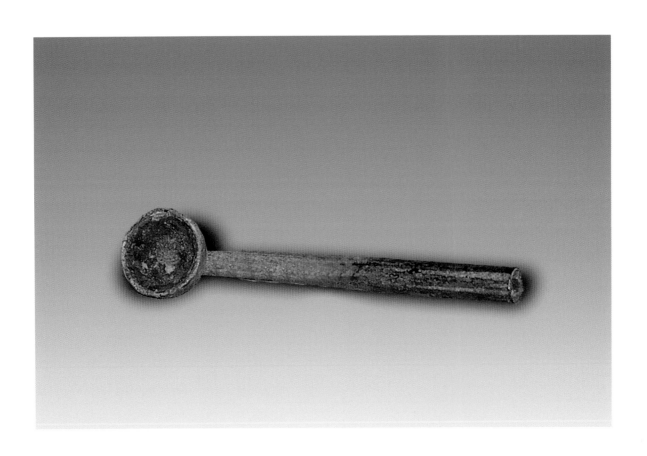

铜烟袋锅

民国时期

铜质

烟锅口径 2 厘米，通长 9.5 厘米，重 1 克

空心柄，一端浅勺状。生活用品，烟具。完整无损。

陕西医史博物馆藏

Copper Tobacco Pipe

Republican Period

Copper

Mouth Diameter of the Head of the Pipe 2 cm/
Length 9.5 cm/ Weight 1 g

The pipe has a hollow handle. One end of the pipe is shaped like a shallow spoon. It is a well-preserved life utensil and was used as a smoking set.

Preserved in Shaanxi Museum of Medical History

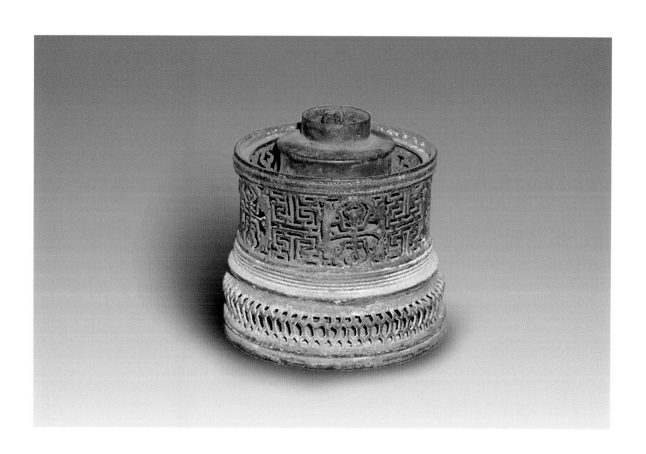

铜烟灯

Copper Tobacco Burner

近代

铜质

口径 7 厘米，底径 8 厘米，通高 7.4 厘米，重
250 克

烟具。完整无损。

陕西医史博物馆藏

Modern Times

Copper

Mouth Diameter 7 cm/Bottom Diameter 8 cm/

Height 7.4 cm/ Weight 250 g

It was used as a smoking set and remains intact.

Preserved in Shaanxi Museum of Medical History

索 引

(馆藏地按拼音字母排序)

北京御生堂中医药博物馆

御生堂药臼、药杵 / 020

药臼 / 022

御生堂金锅铜铲 / 024

御生堂药酒壶 / 056

御生堂针具 / 082

炼丹炉 / 268

北京中医药大学中医药博物馆

中医外科用具 / 090

"午时茶"模具 / 380

成都中医药大学中医药传统文化博物馆

臼 / 026

药臼 / 030

勺 / 062

匙 / 063

匕 / 064

柳叶刀 / 122

温酒器 / 198

盆 / 214

盆 / 216

佛手 / 259

熏炉 / 260

熏炉 / 262

熏炉 / 264

熏炉 / 266

杵臼 / 332

臼 / 334

药臼 / 338

药碾船 / 341

刀 / 343

药罐 / 350

药盒 / 351

药瓶 / 376

熬药罐 / 378

药鼓 / 384

药鼓 / 386

药鼓 / 388

药鼓 / 394

刀 / 396

刀 / 397

刀 / 398

刀 / 399

针 / 402

针 / 403

针 / 404

镊子 / 405

剪 / 406

针筒 / 407

温灸器 / 414

灸条夹 / 415

佩饰 / 416

佩饰 / 417

匙 / 424

匙 / 425

匙 / 426

匙 / 427

勺 / 428

匙 / 429

洗 / 432

唾盂 / 437

唾盂 / 438

唾盂 / 440

灭蚊灯 / 444

酒瓶 / 453

故宫博物院

太医院药锅 / 049

太医院双耳药筛 / 050

太医院盖碗药筛 / 052

御药房温药壶 / 054

金嵌珠翠耳挖勺簪 / 237

江苏省中医药博物馆

串铃 / 002

手术器具 / 091

锡罐 / 190

焦易堂半身铜像 / 310

鼻箔管 / 382

伦敦科学博物馆

中医外科器械 / 093

山东省文物总店

画珐琅人物纹烟壶 / 296

陕西医史博物馆

串铃 / 004

圆铁铃 / 010

铜药臼 / 011

铁药臼 / 012

铁药臼 / 013

铜药臼 / 014

铜药臼 / 016

药锤 / 017

铁药碾槽 / 036

小碾槽 / 037

小铁刀 / 042

小铁刀 / 043

铁药刀 / 044

铁药钳 / 047

铁锻药钳 / 048

铜药匙 / 058

铜药勺头 / 060

铜半圆药瓶 / 065

铜扁药瓶 / 072

铜药盒 / 080

外科手术器械 / 084

中医外科器械 / 087

外科器具 / 088

秤 / 186

铁刀 / 187

铜铲 / 188

铜壶 / 192

铜杯 / 202

铜酒杯 / 203

小铜勺 / 206

铁像 / 207

铜像 / 208

铜盆 / 209

铜盆 / 212

铁盆 / 218

圆铁盒 / 220

圆铁盒 / 222

铁盒 / 224

银帕架 / 226

铜镜 / 227

铜镜 / 228

铜发钗 / 234

铜二须 / 238

银三须 / 239

银三须 / 240

银三须 / 242

银五须 / 244

铜手炉 / 256

铁云牌 / 274

铁磬 / 276

铁灯 / 278

铁灯 / 282

铜灯 / 286

铜鼻烟壶 / 294

小铜鸽子像 / 302

铜币 / 304

铜印（复制）/ 308

铜药臼 / 337

小铁药碾 / 340

铁碾槽 / 342

铁药刀 / 344

铜药匙 / 346

铜药勺 / 347

铜药勺 / 348

铜药勺 / 349

铜膏药刀 / 395

针灸铜人 / 410

拔火罐 / 412

锡罐 / 418

锡火锅 / 420

铜酒杯 / 421

小锡壶 / 422

铜勺 / 430

铜马勺 / 431

铜叉 / 434

景泰蓝小蓝瓶 / 442

铜铃 / 446

铜铃（甩子）/ 447

铁钟 / 448

铜镰 / 450

铜镰 / 451

铜镰 / 452

铜水烟袋 / 455

铜烟袋锅 / 460

铜烟灯 / 461

上海中医药博物馆

铜药臼 / 018

铜碾药船 / 039

铜切药刀 / 046

双桃锡酒壶 / 197

八角铜手炉 / 258

铜灭蚊灯 / 292

中央国医馆徽章 / 320

上海中医专科学校证章 / 322

北京协和医院建院纪念章 / 324

"女子产科学校"印章 / 327

"太乙神针"铜藏针筒 / 408

张雅宗

铁质小针、刀、铜匙 / 094

清宫御用鎏金耳挖勺 / 235

银九针 / 400

中国国家博物馆

太医院药臼、杵 / 019

太医院药碾 / 038

百子图镜 / 231

嘉庆慎思堂十二生肖柄镜 / 233

中国体育博物馆

蹴鞠图漆绘铜牌 / 271

手柄铜斧 / 272

中国箸文化陈列馆

铜箸 / 204

中华医学会 / 上海中医药大学医史博物馆

铜串铃 / 006

铜串铃 / 008

带杵药臼 / 028

带杵药臼 / 032

铜药臼 / 034

碾药船 / 040

链环药瓶 / 066

长颈扁药瓶 / 069

铜药瓶 / 070

麝香银盒 / 074

药盒 / 076

药盒 / 078

外科斜刃刀 / 096

外科斜刃刀 / 098

外科斜刃刀 / 100

外科斜刃刀 / 102

外科斜刃刀 / 104

外科斜刃刀 / 106

外科斜刃刀 / 108

外科斜刃刀 / 110

外科斜刃刀 / 112

外科斜刃刀 / 114

外科斜刃刀 / 116

外科斜刃刀 / 118

外科斜刃刀 / 120

外科弯刃刀 / 124

外科弯刃刀 / 126

外科弯刃刀 / 128

外科弯刃刀 / 130

外科弯刃刀 / 132

外科弯刃刀 / 134

外科弯刃刀 / 136

外科圆刃铲刀 / 138

外科圆刃铲刀 / 140

外科圆刃铲刀 / 142

外科圆刃铲刀 / 144

外科尖刀 / 146

外科尖刀 / 148

外科钩镰刀 / 150

外科钩镰刀 / 152

外科钩镰刀 / 154

外科钩镰刀 / 156

外科两用器 / 158

外科簇尖刺锥 / 160

外科簇尖刺锥 / 162

外科簇尖刺锥 / 164

外科簇尖刺锥 / 166

外科簇尖刺锥 / 168

外科簇尖刺锥 / 170

外科簇尖刺锥 / 172

外科斜刃刀 / 174

外科簇尖刺锥 / 176

外科簇尖刺锥 / 178

外科簇尖刺锥 / 180

外科尖棱锥 / 182

外科尖棱锥 / 184

铝参壶 / 194

铝茶壶 / 200

铜刻花匜 / 211

清理耳鼻工具 / 246

清理耳鼻工具 / 248

剃刀 / 250

指甲套 / 252

指甲套 / 254

油灯盏 / 280

油灯盏座 / 284

铜油灯 / 289

铝台灯 / 290

水烟筒 / 299

烟枪头 / 301

许浚像 / 306

傅连暲墨盒 / 312

陆坤豪挂号牌 / 314

陆坤豪挂号牌 / 316

中华医学会徽章 / 318

上海牙医师公会铜印 / 328

上海牙医师公会铜印 / 330

药盒 / 352

药盒 / 354

药盒 / 356

药盒 / 358

药盒 / 360

药盒 / 362

药盒 / 364

药盒 / 366

药盒 / 368

药盒 / 370

药盒 / 372

药盒 / 374

喷药粉器 / 390

喷药粉器 / 392

烟嘴 / 456

旱烟管 / 458

Index

Chinese Medicine Museum of Beijing Yu Sheng Tang Drugstore

Medicine Mortar with Pestle of Yu Sheng Tang Drugstore / 020

Medicine Mortar / 022

Gold Pot and Bronze Shovel of Yu Sheng Tang Drugstore / 024

Medical Wine Pot of Yu Sheng Tang / 056

Acupuncture Needles from Yu Sheng Tang Drugstore / 082

Alchemy Furnace / 268

Museum of Chinese Medicine, Beijing University of Chinese Medicine

Traditional Chinese Surgical Instruments / 090

"Wu Shi Cha" (Herbal Tea) Mould / 380

Museum of Traditional Chinese Medicine Culture, Chengdu University of Traditional Chinese Medicine

Mortar / 026

Medicine Mortar / 030

Spoon / 062

Spoon / 063

An Ancient Type of Spoon / 064

Lancet (Liu Ye Dao) / 122

Utensil for Heating Wine / 198

Basin / 214

Basin / 216

Censer in the Shape of Fingered Citron / 259

Censer / 260

Censer / 262

Censer / 264

Censer / 266

Mortar with Pestle / 332

Mortar / 334

Medicinal Mortar / 338

Ship-like Medicinal Crusher / 341

Knife / 343

Gallipot / 350

Medicine Box / 351

Medicine Bottles / 376

The Pot for Decocting Herbal Medicine / 378

Drum-like Medical Instrument / 384

Drum-like Medical Instrument / 386

Drum-like Medical Instrument / 388

Drum-like Medical Instrument / 394

Knife / 396

Knife / 397

Knife / 398

Knife / 399

Needle / 402

Needle / 403

Needle / 404

Tweezers / 405

Scissors / 406

Syringe / 407

Moxa Burner / 414

Clamp for Moxa Stick / 415

Accessory / 416

Accessory / 417

Spoon / 424

Spoon / 425

Spoon / 426

Spoon / 427

Spoon / 428

Spoon / 429

Washer / 432

Spittoon / 437

Spittoon / 438

Spittoon / 440

Mosquito Killer Lamp / 444

Wine Bottle / 453

The Palace Museum

Medicine Cauldron of Imperial Hospital / 049

Two-Handle Medicine Sieve of Imperial Hospital / 050

Medicine Sieve Bowl with Cover of Imperial Hospital / 052

Medicine Heating Pot of Imperial Pharmacy / 054

Gold Ear-picker Hairpin Inlaid with Pearl and Jadeite / 237

Jiangsu Museum of Traditional Chinese Medicine

Ring-like Bell / 002

Surgical Instruments / 091

Tin Can / 190

Half-Length Copper Statue of Jiao Yitang / 310

Nasal Tube Covered with Foil / 382

Science Museum, London

Traditional Chinese Surgical Instruments / 093

Shandong Antique Store

Snuff Bottle with Enamel Figure Painting / 296

Shaanxi Museum of Medical History

Ring-like Bell / 004

Round Iron Bell / 010

Copper Medicine Mortar / 011

Iron Medicine Mortar / 012

Iron Medicine Mortar / 013

Copper Medicine Mortar / 014

Copper Medicine Mortar / 016

Medicine Hammer / 017

Iron Medicine Mill Groove / 036

Small Mill Groove / 037

Small Iron Knife / 042

Small Iron Knife / 043

Iron Medical Knife / 044

Iron Medicine Tong / 047

Iron-forged Medicine Tong / 048

Copper Medicine Spoon / 058

Head of Copper Medicine Spoon / 060

Copper Semicircular Medicine Bottle / 065

Copper Flattened Medicine Bottle / 072

Copper Medicine Box / 080

Surgical Instruments / 084

Traditional Chinese Surgical Instruments / 087

Surgical Instruments / 088

Scale / 186

Iron Knife / 187

Copper Shovel / 188

Copper Pot / 192

Copper Cup / 202

Copper Wine Cup / 203

Small Copper Spoon / 206

Iron Statue / 207

Copper Statue / 208

Copper Basin / 209

Copper Basin / 212

Iron Basin / 218

Round Iron Container / 220

Round Iron Container / 222

Iron Container / 224

Silver Handkerchief Holder / 226

Copper Mirror / 227

Copper Mirror / 228

Copper Hairpin / 234

Copper Whisker-like Tools of Two Pieces / 238

Silver Whisker-like Tools of Three Pieces / 239

Silver Whisker-like Tools of Three Pieces / 240

Silver Whisker-like Tools of Three Pieces / 242

Silver Whisker-like Tools of Five Pieces / 244

Copper Handwarmer / 256

Iron "Yun-pai" / 274

Iron "Qing" / 276

Iron Lamp / 278

Iron Lamp / 282

Copper Lamp / 286

Copper Snuff Bottle / 294

Small Copper Pigeon / 302

Copper Coin / 304

Copper Seal (Copy) / 308

Copper Medicinal Mortar / 337

Small Iron Medicinal Crusher / 340

Iron Mill Groove / 342

Iron Medicinal Knife / 344

Copper Medicinal Spoon / 346

Copper Medicinal Ladle / 347

Copper Medicinal Ladle / 348

Copper Medicinal Ladle / 349

Copper Medical Plaster Knife / 395

Copper Acupuncture Status / 410

Cupping Glass / 412

Tin Pot / 418

Tin Stove / 420

Copper Wine Cup / 421

Small Tin Pot / 422

Copper Spoon / 430

Copper Ladle / 431

Copper Fork / 434

Small Cloisonne Vase / 442

Copper Bell / 446

Copper Bell (Hollow Swage) / 447

Iron Bell / 448

Copper Sickle / 450

Copper Sickle / 451

Copper Sickle / 452

Copper Hookah / 455

Copper Tobacco Pipe / 460

Copper Tobacco Burner / 461

Shanghai Museum of Traditional Chinese Medicine

Copper Medicine Mortar / 018

Ship-like Copper Medicine Mill / 039
Copper Knife for Slicing Medicine / 046
Tin Flagon in the Shape of Two Peaches / 197
Octagon Copper Handwarmer / 258
Copper Mosquito-Killing Lamp / 292
Badges of the Central State Hospital / 320
Badge of Shanghai Traditional Chinese Medicine Specialized School / 322
Establishment Souvenir Badge of the Peking Union Medical College Hospital / 324
Seal of the Female Obstetrics School / 327
Copper Cylinder of "Taiyi Miraculous Needles" / 408

Zhang Yazong

Iron Needles, Knife and Copper Spoon / 094
Imperial Gilding Ear Pick / 235
Silver "Nine Needles" / 400

National Museum of China

Medicine Mortar and Pestle of Imperial Hospital / 019
Medicine Mill of Imperial Hospital / 038
Mirror with Children Patterns / 231
Mirror of Severance Hall Made in Jiaqing Periods, with Chinese Zodiac Patterns / 233

China Sports Museum

Lacquered Bronze Plate with Cuju Painting / 271
Copper Axe with Handle / 272

China Chopsticks Culture Museum

Copper Chopsticks / 204

Chinese Medical Association/Museum of Chinese Medicine, Shanghai University of Traditional Chinese Medicine

Copper Ring-like Bell / 006
Copper Ring-like Bell / 008
Medicine Mortar with Pestle / 028
Medicine Mortar with Pestle / 032
Copper Medicine Mortar / 034
Ship-like Medicine Mill / 040
Medicine Bottles Connected with Hinges / 066
Flattened Medicine Bottle with a Long Neck / 069
Coppery Medicine Bottle / 070
Silver Box for Musk / 074
Medicine Box / 076
Medicine Box / 078
Surgical Scalpel with Oblique Blade / 096
Surgical Scalpel with Oblique Blade / 098
Surgical Scalpel with Oblique Blade / 100
Surgical Scalpel with Oblique Blade / 102
Surgical Scalpel with Oblique Blade / 104
Surgical Scalpel with Oblique Blade / 106
Surgical Scalpel with Oblique Blade / 108
Surgical Scalpel with Oblique Blade / 110
Surgical Scalpel with Oblique Blade / 112
Surgical Scalpel with Oblique Blade / 114
Surgical Scalpel with Oblique Blade / 116
Surgical Scalpel with Oblique Blade / 118
Surgical Scalpel with Oblique Edge / 120
Surgical Knife with Curving Edge / 124
Surgical Knife with Curving Edge / 126
Surgical Knife with Curving Edge / 128
Surgical Knife with Curving Edge / 130

Surgical Knife with Curving Edge / 132

Surgical Knife with Curving Edge / 134

Surgical Knife with Curving Edge / 136

Surgical Scraper Knife with Round Edge / 138

Surgical Scraper Knife with Round Edge / 140

Surgical Scraper Knife with Round Edge / 142

Surgical Scraper Knife with Round Edge / 144

Surgical Sharp Knife / 146

Surgical Sharp Knife / 148

Surgical Sickle-like Knife with Hook / 150

Surgical Sickle-like Knife with Hook / 152

Surgical Sickle-like Knife with Hook / 154

Surgical Sickle-like Knife with Hook / 156

Surgical Appliance of Two-Purpose / 158

Surgical Awl with Pointed Tip / 160

Surgical Awl with Pointed Tip / 162

Surgical Awl with Pointed Tip / 164

Surgical Awl with Pointed Tip / 166

Surgical Awl with Pointed Tip / 168

Surgical Awl with Pointed Tip / 170

Surgical Awl with Pointed Tip / 172

Surgical Knife with Oblique Edge / 174

Surgical Awl with Pointed Tip / 176

Surgical Awl with Pointed Tip / 178

Surgical Awl with Pointed Tip / 180

Surgical Awl with Sharp and Pyramid-Shaped Tip / 182

Surgical Awl with Sharp and Pyramid-Shaped Tip / 184

Aluminum Pot for Cooking Ginseng Soup / 194

Aluminum Tea Pot / 200

Copper Gourd-shaped Ladle with Engraved Designs / 211

A Nose and Ear Cleaning Tool / 246

A Nose and Ear Cleaning Tool / 248

Shaver / 250

Fingernail Cover / 252

Fingernail Cover / 254

Oil Lamp / 280

Oil Lamp Pedestal / 284

Copper Oil Lamp / 289

Aluminum Table Lamp / 290

Chinese Water Pipe / 299

Smoking Pipe Head / 301

Statue of Xu Jun / 306

Fu Lianzhang's Ink Box / 312

Registration Tablet of Lu Kunhao / 314

Registration Tablet of Lu Kunhao / 316

Badges of the Chinese Medical Association / 318

Copper Seal of Shanghai Dentist Association / 328

Copper Seal of Shanghai Dental Association / 330

Medicine Box / 352

Medicine Box / 354

Medicine Box / 356

Medicine Box / 358

Medicine Box / 360

Medicine Box / 362

Medicine Box / 364

Medicine Box / 366

Medicine Box / 368

Medicine Box / 370

Medicine Box / 372

Medicine Box / 374

Medical Spray Tube / 390

Medical Spray Tube / 392

Tobacco Pipe / 456

Tobacco Pipe / 458

参考文献

[1] 李经纬 . 中国古代医史图录 [M]. 北京：人民卫生出版社，1992.

[2] 傅维康，李经纬，林昭庚 . 中国医学通史：文物图谱卷 [M]. 北京：人民卫生出版社，2000.

[3] 和中浚，吴鸿洲 . 中华医学文物图集 [M]. 成都：四川人民出版社，2001.

[4] 上海中医药博物馆 . 上海中医药博物馆馆藏珍品 [M]. 上海：上海科学技术出版社，2013.

[5] 西藏自治区博物馆 . 西藏博物馆 [M]. 北京：五洲传播出版社，2005.

[6] 崔乐泉 . 中国古代体育文物图录：中英文本 [M]. 北京：中华书局，2000.

[7] 张金明，陆雪春 . 中国古铜镜鉴赏图录 [M]. 北京：中国民族摄影艺术出版社，2002.

[8] 文物精华编辑委员会 . 文物精华 [M]. 北京：文物出版社，1964.

[9] 谭维四 . 湖北出土文物精华 [M]. 武汉：湖北教育出版社，2001.

[10] 常州市博物馆 . 常州文物精华 [M]. 北京：文物出版社，1998.

[11] 镇江博物馆 . 镇江文物精华 [M]. 合肥：黄山书社，1997.

[12] 贵州省文化厅，贵州省博物馆 . 贵州文物精华 [M]. 贵阳：贵州人民出版社，2005.

[13] 徐良玉 . 扬州馆藏文物精华 [M]. 南京：江苏古籍出版社，2001.

[14] 昭陵博物馆，陕西历史博物馆 . 昭陵文物精华 [M]. 西安：陕西人民美术出版社，1991.

[15] 南通博物苑 . 南通博物苑文物精华 [M]. 北京：文物出版社，2005.

[16] 邯郸市文物研究所 . 邯郸文物精华 [M]. 北京：文物出版社，2005.

[17] 张秀生，刘友恒，聂连顺，等 . 中国河北正定文物精华 [M]. 北京：文化艺术出版社，1998.

[18] 陕西省咸阳市文物局 . 咸阳文物精华 [M]. 北京：文物出版社，2002.

[19] 安阳市文物管理局 . 安阳文物精华 [M]. 北京：文物出版社，2004.

[20] 深圳市博物馆 . 深圳市博物馆文物精华 [M]. 北京：文物出版社，1998.

[21]《中国文物精华》编辑委员会 . 中国文物精华（1993）[M]. 北京：文物出版社，1993.

[22] 夏路，刘永生 . 山西省博物馆馆藏文物精华 [M]. 太原：山西人民出版社，1999.

[23] 文物精华编辑委员会 . 文物精华 [M]. 文物出版社，1957.

[24] 山西博物院，湖北省博物馆 . 荆楚长歌：九连墩楚墓出土文物精华 [M]. 太原：山西人民出版社，2011.

[25] 刘广堂，石金鸣，宋建忠 . 晋国雄风：山西出土两周文物精华 [M]. 沈阳：万卷出版公司，2009.

[26] 沈君山，王国平，单迎红 . 滦平博物馆馆藏文物精华 [M]. 北京：中国文联出版社，2012.

[27] 张家口市博物馆 . 张家口市博物馆馆藏文物精华 [M]. 北京：科学出版社，2011.

[28] 浙江省文物考古研究所 . 浙江考古精华 [M]. 北京：文物出版社，1999.

[29] 故宫博物院 . 故宫雕刻珍萃 [M]. 北京：紫禁城出版社，2004.

[30] 故宫博物院紫禁城出版社 . 故宫博物院藏宝录 [M]. 上海：上海文艺出版社，1986.

[31] 首都博物馆 . 大元三都 [M]. 北京：科学出版社，2016.

[32] 新疆维吾尔自治区博物馆 . 新疆出土文物 [M]. 北京：文物出版社，1975.

[33] 王兴伊，段逸山 . 新疆出土涉医文书辑校 [M]. 上海：上海科学技术出版社，2016.

[34] 刘学春 . 刍议医药卫生文物的概念与分类标准 [J]. 中华中医药杂志，2016，31（11）:4406-4409.

[35] 上海古籍出版社 . 中国艺海 [M]. 上海：上海古籍出版社，1994.

[36] 紫都，岳鑫 . 一生必知的 200 件国宝 [M]. 呼和浩特：远方出版社，2005.

[37] 谭维四 . 湖北出土文物精华 [M]. 武汉：湖北教育出版社，2001.

[38] 张建青 . 青海彩陶收藏与鉴赏 [M]. 北京：中国文史出版社，2007.

[39] 银景琦 . 仡佬族文物 [M]. 南宁：广西人民出版社，2014.

[40] 廖果，梁峻，李经纬 . 东西方医学的反思与前瞻 [M]. 北京：中医古籍出版社，2002.

[41] 梁峻，张志斌，廖果，等 . 中华医药文明史集论 [M]. 北京：中医古籍出版社，2003.

[42] 郑蓉，庄乾竹，刘聪，等 . 中国医药文化遗产考论 [M]. 北京：中医古籍出版社，2005.